Fatass No More!
How I Lost Weight and Still Ate Cheeseburgers and Fries

Also by Kim Rinehart:

The Big Clean: How to Organize Your Pad and Free Your Mind

Fatass No More!

How I Lost Weight and Still Ate Cheeseburgers and Fries

By

Kim Rinehart

Bright Yellow Hat

Fatass No More! How I Lost Weight and Still Ate Cheeseburgers
and Fries
By
Kim Rinehart

Bright Yellow Hat
an imprint of New Tradition Books
ISBN 1932420134

For information contact:
Bright Yellow Hat
brightyellowhat@yahoo.com

For the dieters.

Contents

Diets suck.

Let's face the facts—diets suck. They force us to change our natural eating patterns and that's why they suck. And they're always too good to be true, aren't they? They claim you can lose an extraordinary amount of weight in no time flat. They claim this and they claim that and most of them never keep their promises.

This is not a diet.

What if I told you there is an easy way to lose weight and it doesn't cost one red cent? What if I told you that you can do it on your own and that you can even eat cheeseburgers and French fries while you're doing it? What if I told you that you can do it without starving yourself and that all you have to do is a little rearranging of your eating habits? What if I told you that you will never have to go on another diet in your life and still be able to maintain your weight?

I know what you're thinking: "She's going to tell me how to lose weight by eating cheeseburgers and fries? I've heard it all now! Why did I even pick this book up? This is crazy!"

No, it isn't. But diets are.

And they don't work. They never have and they never, ever will. It usually goes a little something like this: You diet, you lose a little weight, you stop dieting, you gain back more weight. It's an endless cycle of counting calories and watching everything you put into your mouth and it just makes your head hurt, doesn't it? God only knows what you've done and how much money you've spent doing it. I know I did a lot and there was only one thing that ever worked for me. I stopped dieting.

Yup. You heard me.

I just stopped dieting. I hated it anyway and it never did me any good. Why torture myself? And that's all you're doing too. You're looking for a secret, magical way to shed those pounds and, folks, there isn't any. There is no magic pill or any big secret to losing weight. There is, however, a huge industry that will tell you otherwise, but that's a different topic for a different day.

So, what can you do if you just can't seem to shed those pounds? What can you do if you've tried everything and everything didn't work? Here's an idea: Don't go on a diet!

Radical? Hardly. Diets fail because they wreak havoc on your body by forcing it into the survival zone. They also fail because diets are an unnatural way to eat.

No big secret: You have to eat. Big secret: You can't eat everything you want. Bigger secret: You can eat what you want most of the time. Biggest secret: You can only do it about once a day.

Don't get confused just yet. Let me break it down for you, starting with the love of my two favorite food items.

To me, there is nothing like a cheeseburger and fries. And I mean *nothing*. Which would I prefer? A fancy meal in a fancy restaurant or a cheeseburger and fries? You got it. Cheeseburgers and fries are my cake and I like to eat them— a lot. Just the thought of a delicious burger topped with cheese and hot, steaming French fries are enough to make my mouth water. Add a glass of soda, and I'm good to go.

I don't only just eat cheeseburgers and fries, of course. I also eat pizza, salads, fresh fruits and vegetables, ribs, you name it. I eat what I want and when I want. Mostly.

Sounds crazy, doesn't it? Eating what you want and not gaining weight. How could that be?

Here's the secret: I eat what I want but not every day and certainly not for every meal. Also, I usually only eat these foods for lunch, earlier in the day. That's the trick, that's what's helped me lose weight and that's what kept me from gaining it back. That's what kept me from going crazy and feeling deprived. I'm going to get into more detail a little later on, but right now, let me explain how I got here.

It was this love of cheeseburgers and fries that caused me to gain an awful amount of weight. And I gained it because I overindulged and also because I was on a very hectic and stressful schedule. In addition to that, just like many other Americans, I thought it was my right to consume more food than I needed. *Way more food.* I didn't stop when I was no longer hungry. I didn't stop when I was full. I didn't stop until I thought I was about to burst. And the kicker is, a few hours after I had eaten, I would snack on a candy bar and a soda. The more I ate, the more I wanted to eat.

I overindulged and I paid the price. My weight rose until I was about one-hundred and sixty-five pounds, forty-five pounds heavier than I'd been as a teenager. On a five-foot-three inch frame that spells disaster.

One day, I woke up and knew I had to stop. I realized if I didn't get my weight under control, I never would. That day, I set out to lose the weight and keep it off by using my own method. It was hard but not impossible. And this is what I want to share.

People are always asking me how I stay thin. And I always tell them the same thing—I eat what I want but I don't overindulge. I also eat most of my calories earlier in the day so my body has time to actually burn what I've consumed before I eat again. It's not rocket science, it's just a good way to lose weight, keep it off and not feel deprived when you're doing it.

I will take you step by step into what I did to finally reach my current weight and what I do to keep it off. And this includes exercising, which is always a good idea as it helps a person maintain their weight and makes them feel better, too.

I am not going to tell you what to eat nor am I going to give you recipes you'll never use. I'm just going to tell you what I did and the reasoning behind it. Also, I am not going to call what I do "dieting". Mainly because "dieting" is *not* what I do.

However, you should be aware that the healthier you eat, the healthier you will be. So, when you eat what you like, be sure to mix it up with fresh vegetables and fruits occasionally. But, as I said, I'm not going to tell you what to eat as that's up to you. I can only tell you what I did to lose the weight. *What you put into your mouth is your own business.*

Another thing I'm going to discuss is some of the reasons behind weight gain, and also touch on subjects like binge eating. I am going to include some commentary on why I think people don't lose weight when they should. I will also touch on health issues as well as give tips along the way to help you lose the weight, but more importantly, *keep it off.*

And that's what we're after here. Many people go on diets and lose weight but for the most part, it comes right back. That's the difference between this weight loss plan and diets. If you do this one right, you'll have a much better chance of keeping the weight off. One reason behind this is because you are going to change your eating patterns. You are going to eat whatever you want to eat, but you're just not going to indulge every single day and for every single meal.

I am just an everyday, ordinary person. I know when I was trying to lose weight, it was the stories and struggles of "normal" people that inspired me, not the story of some model or actress who looked liked they just went to a plastic surgeon or had a "team" helping them do it.

I'm not telling you this is the way you should do it. I'm not telling you that you *should* do it. These are only my experiences and my struggles with food and weight gain. I am not a doctor nor am I an "expert". I am just a regular person much like you who struggled for years with my weight. Take what you will but note that all of this is only applicable to my own, personal experiences.

Important note: Before you begin this or any other diet and exercise program, consult your physician.

It's this easy:
My Eat What You Like
Weight Loss Method.

What I do is simple. I just eat most of my calories at lunchtime. For breakfast, I might have a bowl of cereal or a yogurt. For lunch, I eat what I like and I eat until I am satisfied, but not bursting at the seams. For supper, I eat something small like a bowl of cereal or popcorn. And I don't snack. Basically, I watch my portion sizes at breakfast and supper but for lunch, I can eat what I like, *but I don't overindulge.* Also, if I want a cookie, I have a cookie but not everyday or after every meal. The trick is to not deprive yourself of your favorite foods, but to *decrease the amount of food you're eating.* This way, your body has a chance to catch up with the calories you've previously stored and burn them. That's what makes you lose weight.

So, before we go any further, I am going to go over every detail of what I do to stay thin. This way, you're not skimming the chapters and trying to figure it out. It's loud and clear right here.

This is how it works:

- ✓ Admit to yourself that you're overweight.
- ✓ Find the desire to lose the weight. Tap into why you want to do it and why you need to do it.
- ✓ Make a vow to stop dieting.
- ✓ Eat what you like.
- ✓ Gradually—*gradually!*—decrease your food intake.
- ✓ The "eat what you like" plan is simple: Have a light breakfast, a moderate lunch, then top it off with a light supper. I find that eating my "big" meal earlier in the day gives my body time to catch up and burn the calories I previously stored.
- ✓ Gradually stop snacking.
- ✓ Desserts are usually just habits. Skip them a few times and you'll be surprised at how your desire for them will decrease.
- ✓ However, if you want a cookie or whatever, have one *but only one*. And try not to eat a cookie everyday.
- ✓ Begin a light exercise program.
- ✓ Eat slowly.
- ✓ A few months into this, you will ask yourself how you consumed all that food in the first place.
- ✓ Watch out for triggers that cause binge eating: Depression, PMS, stress, boredom, et al.
- ✓ Watch out for food and restaurant commercials and advertisements. These lovely images on the TV do make the saliva run. Learn to ignore.
- ✓ When you find yourself craving a snack or extra helping of food, ask yourself if you're really hungry or just eating to be eating.
- ✓ Overeating is sometimes just a habit and you do it just to be doing it. Break this habit!

- ✓ Buy a scale and *weigh every single day*. This will help you keep track of what you're losing. If you're not losing anything, it will let you know that you need to cut back more.
- ✓ Don't eat because of imagined "weakness" or "tiredness". These two things are the biggest causes of weight gain. If you feel "weak" or "tired" all the time, consult your physician. (Some people mistake being tired for being hungry and think if they eat, they won't be tired anymore. Most times, it makes them *more* tired.)
- ✓ Set weight loss goals of less than twenty pounds. Once you lose the twenty pounds, set another goal, maybe this time going for ten or fifteen. And so on and so forth until you've reached the weight you are most comfortable with and that is about right for your height.
- ✓ Understand that you *will* hit a weight loss plateau. This is normal. When this happens, ask yourself if this is good enough and if not, ask yourself what one food you can cut out to get the extra pounds off.
- ✓ Don't blame anyone for your weight. You alone are responsible for it.
- ✓ Drink about eight glasses of water a day.
- ✓ If you drink alcoholic beverages, try cutting them down. Drinking everyday keeps weight on you. Remember, if you put it in your body, you are going to have to burn it off.
- ✓ Keep in mind that in order to lose weight, you will have to be a little hungry. A little hungry does not mean starving, though.
- ✓ Consult your physician before you begin this or any weight loss program.

The best part of this weight loss plan is that it's really easy to maintain. All you have to do is to continue to eat like this. By cutting back on your food intake, you're changing your eating patterns forever, not just for a few months. Soon, you'll want less and less food and it will become like second nature to not eat as much.

Could it be that simple? Is it that easy? Yes, it is. Read on to find out more.

This is what you do each day.

- ✓ **For breakfast:** Eat lightly. Have a bowl of cereal—preferably something high in fiber—or oatmeal or a piece of fruit or an egg on toast. Sometime small, though. Not a three egg omelet and certainly not a stack of pancakes with syrup. Eat what you like, just not a lot of it. Leave yourself a little hungry but not staving.
- ✓ **For lunch:** Eat what you like—food that you would normally have for lunch, not a chocolate cake or anything like that. This is your meal of the day and treat it as such. Order what you want, however, only eat until you are satisfied and *not stuffed.*
- ✓ **For supper:** Have steamed veggies or a bowl of cereal or a few chicken strips, or a bowl of popcorn or whatever you like. It's up to you but remember this is a small meal, not something huge. Eat something small but good that will get you though the night. Leave yourself slightly hungry.
- ✓ **Drink either water or juice with your meals.** (Drink at least eight glasses of water a day.)
- ✓ **Do not snack at all.** If you have to snack, snack on something like celery or pickles or carrots or a handful of microwave popcorn. No crackers and no potato chips and no cookies and certainly no candy bars.

✓ *If you must have a dessert* after one of your meals, buy whatever you like—a bag of cookies or snack sized candy bars—and have *only* one. Only one. Tomorrow, if you like, you can have another one. *But not until tomorrow.*

✓ *Vary your food each day.* This way, you're not feeling deprived.

✓ *Watch your alcoholic beverages.* Maybe only drink on the weekend.

✓ *Do not leave yourself starving!* If you do this, you will only binge.

You have to understand that you are relearning yourself how to eat. It doesn't matter what you eat as long as you eat *smaller amounts.* Obviously, the healthier you eat, the healthier you will be. I am not emphasizing eating only junk food and I do suggest that you mix it up with fruits and veggies.

The basic idea is to eat what you like, but just don't overdo it. Also, eat most of your calories earlier in the day. If you are in the habit of eating two big meals a day—one for lunch and one for supper—then the goal is to cut out supper and replace it with a smaller meal. The point is to gradually cut down on your food consumption until your appetite wanes.

Keep in mind that in order to lose any weight, you have to be hungry. Of course, this doesn't mean starving where you might risk getting light-headed and dizzy. As I've said, by eating most of your calories around lunch, you are giving your body a chance to catch up with all the calories you've consumed and burn them. That's what it's mostly about—you have to burn more calories than you consume in a day in order to lose weight. It's simple mathematics when you get right down to it. Calories are calories and if you ingest a calorie, it has to be burned off in order to lose weight. Mostly, you are allowing your body to play catch-up with the overindulgences of the past.

Overeating is a habit that was learned. All you're doing now is overwriting it with a new habit.

This is not hard. Losing weight does not have to be hard. Don't make it hard. It's not impossible. Just start today and you will lose the weight. It will take time and effort. You will have to watch how much you eat and if you overeat, you will have to eat a little less the next day to make up for it. Breaking that habit of overeating is what you're after. If you can do this, you can win the battle of the bulge.

I will make suggestions throughout the book about maintaining your weight once you get it off and there's a short chapter at the end, but here's a brief note: Because you have changed your eating patterns and have stopped snacking and overeating, all you have to do is to maintain that. Of course, you can never go back to eating the amount of food that you once ate. (And why would you want to?) All you have to do now is have your three meals a day: One small breakfast, one moderate lunch and one small supper. That's it. If you continue this, you really shouldn't have to even worry about weight gain. Also, you'll have a little more flexibility about what/when/how you eat, but the idea of the plan stays the same. Keep an eye on the scale, too. It's what's going to help you know when you gain a few pounds and when you do, all you have to do is cut back on your food intake.

This is my story.

The first step to losing weight is admitting you are overweight. I had to do it and it was hard. Nevertheless, it took about a year to admit I was gaining weight. I mean, I knew I was overweight but I was too lazy and too in denial to do anything about it.

After I got married, I started eating everything in the world that I wanted to eat. Yum, yum, yum. Food—I just loved food! I also stopped caring what I looked like. What did it matter anyway? I was married and wasn't worried anymore about "getting a man". I'd done that already and now I could relax and just be myself.

I noticed that I really started to put on the pounds when I took a job as a photographer. It was my first professional job and required a lot of long distance travel and a lot of nights sleeping in hotel rooms alone. The only thing I enjoyed about that job was the food. I got a daily meal allowance and used it to the best of my advantage.

As I've said, I loved to eat. Still do. There is nothing like food to make a person feel good, is there? Being out on the road with a big food allowance allowed me to indulge, or shall I say, *over*indulge. I could eat just about anything I wanted. And whenever I wanted. I had plenty of time at night alone and there was nothing to do *but* eat.

For instance, I would have a sausage and egg biscuit for breakfast. For lunch, I might have pizza and salad, or my old favorite, cheeseburger and fries. For supper, I could afford a steak and potato and usually a dessert of some sort.

But not only was I eating three huge meals a day, I was also snacking. Whenever I got my breaks, I would get a bag of popcorn or a candy bar, complete with a soda. My world began to revolve around food. All I thought about was when I'd eat and what I'd eat. I ate and ate and ate. I was eating enough for a third world country. I didn't need this much food but because I was lonely and working so hard, I thought I deserved *something*. Food was my something.

I had been doing this for about six months and knew I needed to cut back. I didn't weigh myself or anything, but I knew I was getting heavier because my clothes kept getting tighter and tighter. So, when I had supper, I would go for salads. Well, I tried to. I am just not a big salad eater and never have been. When I would pull up to the drive-thru, I would long for a cheeseburger. So, I would get a salad *and* a cheeseburger. And a soda and why not a few fries, too? At least I was getting my vegetables. After I did this a few times, I knew it was useless, so I stopped eating salads.

After about two years of eating like a pig—I mean, being a photographer—I took a job in a daycare. There we had an on-site cook who prepared all kinds of delicious foods. We had two big meals a day—breakfast and lunch— and I was expected to sit at the little tables and eat with the kids "family style," which means we had plates and bowls on the table. This was to help the kids learn how to use utensils and serve themselves. This was a learning process for them. For me, it was a way to pack on more pounds because I was not only eating two big meals at the daycare, but on most days, I would go home and eat a big supper too. In addition to that, it was *always* someone's birthday, and we usually had cake and chips and soda in celebration.

It did occur to me that I was gaining weight because I kept buying bigger and bigger sizes and even purchased a few t-shirts that were "one size fits all". But, for some reason, I just thought that was the natural progression of life. Most everyone I knew gained weight once they were married and got a "real" job. And, hey, I was married and had a "real" job now, too.

After about a year at the daycare, I took a job in social services. I continued to eat three meals a day, every single day. Big meals, lots of calories and oh, so good food. I would meet colleagues for breakfast meetings, I'd do lunch on my own, and then I'd go home and eat supper with my husband.

I don't see how I got any work done. All I did was eat!

For some reason, I thought I could eat whatever I wanted, whenever I wanted. I knew I was getting heavier but, because I had always been skinny when I was younger, I just didn't face it. Or, maybe, I thought it was something that couldn't happen to me.

Perhaps the real reason was because I was slightly depressed. My life wasn't really going in the direction I had wanted and I felt bogged down by the "new" responsibility of being married and of being an adult. Food helped me to get though the tough times. It was a way to medicate. Not feeling well today? How about a milkshake? Down and depressed? How about a king-sized candy bar and a soda? So stressed you feel like your head is about to explode? How about some potato chips? But as soon as the food had been swallowed, I went right back to the same-old-same-old. It was a relief, but only temporary.

I ignored it, of course. I mean, I didn't have to deal if I didn't recognize it and I didn't have to deal if I refused to look in the mirror. My husband never said anything to me. Neither did anyone else. No one said, "Damn! You're gaining a lot of weight!" No one says this stuff because it's not polite. It's rude and makes you feel like crap.

I wish someone had said it to me. I went through about five years of gradual weight gain because no one had the nerve to tell me I was getting fat. But then again, I wouldn't have listened to them anyway. I wouldn't have believed it. Me? Fat? *NEVER!* Something would have to hit me like a ton of bricks before I would begin to see the shape my body was in. No one could have told me what was going on. I had to see it for myself. And one day, I did.

After years of ignoring the fact that I was rapidly gaining weight and losing all my self-esteem in the process, I finally did the thing that most of us have to do—I looked in the mirror *and saw what I really looked like*. For the first time in a long time, I saw myself. And I didn't like it one bit.

I was overweight. No, I was fat. *I was fat.* After years of ignoring it and years of pretending to be "okay" with it, it hit me like a ton of bricks.

It came about quite accidentally. I hadn't planned on looking at myself that day. In fact, I never looked in the mirror for too long. I would just give myself a good once-over in the morning and for the rest of the day, I would avoid all mirrors—even my reflection in windows. If I didn't look, I couldn't see. I didn't do this deliberately; it was more of a subconscious thing.

On that fateful day, I walked by a floor-length mirror in my bedroom and glanced into it. For a split second, I thought, "Who is that?" I looked around the room. I was alone. That could only mean...oh, no.

I looked back. Actually, I *forced* myself to look back. Then I jumped away from the mirror. Oh. My God! No. No, no, no and no! That was me! It was me staring back at me with recognition and complete and utter shock.

What the hell happened to me? I was a fatass!

I studied myself. There was something about me that didn't make sense. I mean, I wasn't stupid. I knew I was overweight. Just *how* overweight was another matter. A few extra pounds here or there wasn't a big deal. But there were more than a few now and it was making me look slightly different. So, what *was* different? What was different about me that I hadn't noticed before?

Then I realized what it was. The thing that caught my attention and really took me by surprise wasn't what I thought it would be. It wasn't my big belly or my enormous thighs or my swollen face that made me look twice. *It was my arms!*

Yes, my arms. They say the last place you gain weight will be the first you lose it. Well, I hadn't "noticed" that I had been gaining weight anywhere. So when I caught sight of my arms, I nearly passed out. It had been years since I had given myself a good, honest look in the mirror. What I saw did, in fact, make me cringe.

Because I was home, I had on one of those little baby t-shirts that were popular at the time. Not that I would have worn it out in public, but at home, I'd wear it. What horrified me was the fact that my arms were so big there were rolls of fat hanging under the sleeves of the t-shirt. I shouldn't have even been wearing it! I looked like that baby in the Michelin tire commercial. He's got little rolls of fat on his arms but it's cute. And he's a baby; he can get away with it.

I just stopped, stared at myself and thought, "There is no way I'm that big." Even as I stared at the evidence of my fat, I would not, could *not* admit it.

I almost had a panic attack. There was no way this could have happened to me. Like I said, I knew I was gaining weight, but *that* much? I didn't eat *that* much. There was no way. I had always been skinny and now I was...I was... I had a hard time even saying it to myself, but I was fat.

The only way I could have gained that much weight would be to eat all the time. I didn't eat all the time! In fact, I didn't eat that much at all.

That's when I knew I had a problem and the biggest problem was *admitting to myself that I was overweight.* And the only way to get this overweight would to be to eat a lot. So, I forced myself to think about what I'd eaten that day.

So, what had I eaten that day? First I'd had a soda, then an egg and bacon biscuit. Next I'd eaten lunch with co-workers and we'd had pizza and sweet tea. For supper, I had spaghetti with garlic bread and a soda. Well, I had two sodas at supper. Any snacks? Yeah, I had grabbed a bag of chips at a convenience store with a soda when I stopped for gas. I thought about it and realized that I had also eaten a bag of popcorn later that night while watching TV.

I added the calories up in my head and came up with a figure right at four-thousand calories, if not more. *Four-thousand calories in a single day.* That was probably more than enough food for two people.

Now that knew why I'd gained so much weight—because I'd been eating enough for two people—I had to face my biggest nightmare—the scale. The scale didn't lie and it told me that I weighed one-hundred and sixty-five pounds.

This could not be happening.

Instead of having a complete and total nervous breakdown, I stepped off the scale and told myself that I was not gaining one more pound. Not one more pound. And then I went into my bedroom, stripped down to my underwear and forced myself to look in the mirror again. I was fat everywhere. At least it was pretty evenly distributed,

I reassured myself. But then, I took a closer look. I had back fat! *Back fat!* Rolls of it. I looked hideous. I really did. That much extra weight on my small frame just looked... It looked awful. It really, really did.

I wanted to break down and cry. I wanted to throw things around the room. But I didn't do anything violent. I did something that needed to be done a long time ago. *I accepted it.* But, most importantly, I accepted the fact that I was going to get rid of it. I had to get myself back in shape, some day, some way. I had my fun for years overeating and now it was time to do something about it. I had let myself go and now it was time to find myself. I would be a fatass no more!

But how could I do it? It wasn't that hard putting the weight on, but I knew it would be twice as hard taking it off. I briefly considered just getting liposuction all over my body. But I couldn't afford it. Besides, without changing my eating habits, the fat would have been back in no time. (I know a person who did this. She spent over six-thousand dollars for liposuction and continued to eat the way she had eaten before the operation. Thusly, the operation did her no good and she was right back where she started from. Except this time, she was in debt.)

It didn't matter how I was going to do it. There was a way. There had to be a way to remove this flab from my body. I had done it to myself. No one had force-fed me. No one had tricked me into gaining weight. It was my fault and my responsibility. And I had to do something about it.

And that's when I started to diet.

The diets from hell.

Now let's get to the fun stuff. Here are just a few of the diets I tried in my quest to lose weight. I'd be willing to bet money that you'll recognize some of them.

First of all, I tried the *shakes diet* where you just drink a shake instead of eating a meal. And I got the shakes, literally. They left me so hungry, I had hallucinations about food. Visions of cheeseburgers and milkshakes floated around my head. Of course, all I was eating was one *very* small meal a day and some stuff mixed into a glass of milk. By the end of that diet, I was so hungry, I was eating a meal *while* I drank the shake. I didn't want to waste it, you know? Therefore, this diet accomplished nothing.

Then it was on to the good old *heart patient's diet*. During this diet, I was allowed, I think, about a thousand calories a day. Sometimes I would be so hungry I couldn't see straight. I can't remember the specifics, but I do know I ate a lot of boiled eggs and plain toast, which is always tasty and good. *Not.*

Let's see…the next diet was some kind of *liquid diet*. This diet promised that if I drank some liquid stuff and nothing else for three days, I would miraculously lose about ten pounds. This diet was from hell. My stomach lurched and I felt dizzy all the time because, hey, I wasn't eating anything and my body was pissed off about it. I did lose five pounds, which I immediately gained back when I resumed eating.

Then I heard that carbohydrates are evil, so I went on the *low-carb diet*. No, carbs really aren't evil, but this diet was. It was evil! It sounded like such a good idea at the time. Basically, you cut out most of your carbs—breads, pastas, etc.—and replace with protein. Sounded simple enough and I do love bacon! And I could eat a whole pound of it if I wanted to! Or at least I thought I could. (Did it ever occur to these people that there aren't many people who would *want* to eat a whole pound of freakin' bacon?!) The second day of this I had a terrible headache that stayed with me for the duration of the diet which was two miserable weeks. I also had constipation and I felt tired, weak and dizzy. I did lose five or so pounds. And those five pounds came right back when I quit this diet.

Then I tried some *diet pills*. They revved me up so much I thought my heart was going to come out of my chest. I didn't gain any weight with this fad, but I didn't lose any either. But I did spend about fifty bucks on it.

I did what I like to call the *no-taste diet* where all you eat is canned tuna and boiled eggs—always a lovely combination. I lost four pounds that came right back after I resumed eating something besides tuna and boiled eggs.

I did the *starvation diet* and ate just about nothing for two weeks. I lost about six or so pounds and it came right back when I started to eat again, with one pound added for good measure.

I did the *juice diet* and the *Hollywood diet* and the *idiot diet* and the *"I hate myself"* diet and every diet in the world and *nothing worked!*

Why didn't it work? The reason was because I wasn't eating normally. I was eating like I was in a medical experiment or something. None of the diets made much sense but not doing something was the only other option. So I did every diet I could get my hands on.

This went on for a long time.

It seemed as though the more I dieted, the more confused I became. Carbs are good. No carbs are bad. Fat is good. No! It's bad! Cut out your sugar. A little sugar ain't such a bad thing. Don't eat fruit. Eat lots of fruit. Starve yourself for just three days and you will lose all the weight you want! Stand on your head, stick your fingers in your ears and scream at the top of your lungs, "LA LA LA LA LA!"

And that's what I did in the end. I was almost crazy. These diets weren't working and they were just too hard. If any one of them had been the "miracle" cure they claimed to be, I would have been as skinny as a rail. They were all about deprivation, I realized. It was all about punishment for gaining the weight in the first place. That's what these diets were—punishment for being a bad girl. Sure, I knew what I had put my body though by gaining the weight, but did it have to be this hard? Did it have to be like pulling teeth to lose any amount of weight? Why couldn't it be simpler? Easier? None of it made any sense and none of it worked.

When the diets wouldn't work, I would get so upset. I would spend all this money and all this time looking for something to help me and none of them did. None of them! They were evil! They were the spawn of the devil! They were also very devious, these diets. They told me one thing and if I did it, I would lose weight like *that!* And sometimes I did lose weight just like *that* but it would always come back once I got off the diet.

It seemed as though every single one of these diets failed on all levels. I just wanted *something* to work. I didn't care what it was. I was willing to do anything to lose the weight. *Anything.* And I did try just about everything. And nothing ever worked for very long.

It's like I was setting myself up for failure.

One day I thought about how nice it would to be able to eat anything I wanted and still lose weight. But you can't eat what you want to eat and lose weight. That's what they tell you, isn't it? Don't eat what you want, eat what *they* say. So, there was no way I could eat the foods I loved and lose the pounds.

Or could I?

I hadn't had this epiphany yet, so I kept dieting and the weight wasn't budging. Five pounds here or there wasn't cutting it. It was like I was stuck and nothing I did made me unstuck. I felt like such a loser. I had this huge desire to lose the weight and look good but I didn't know how.

But we do what we're taught, right? If you diet, you will lose weight. So that's what I did. I went from one fad diet to the next looking for the miracle combination that would make me skinny again. I guess I was just too oblivious to realize that if it hadn't worked by then, it wasn't *going* to work. Like I've said, I was doing what I had been taught by everyone to do—diet in order to lose weight. However, I was dieting but I wasn't losing any significant amount of weight.

It was depressing, to say the least. I finally just stopped dieting. I mean, why bother? It wasn't doing me any good. I kept eating, too, but I didn't know not to. Or *how* to, I should say.

One day, however, I sat down and said to myself, "I am sick of doing this. I am trying to lose this weight and I just can't do it. I love good food too much. It should *not* be this hard."

If I could just eat what I wanted, then I would be alright. I didn't like dieting and I hated deprivation. Why not eat what I want but just eat about half of it? And then I thought, "I am going to eat what I want but only at lunch. I can have whatever I want and eat until I am satisfied but then I'll stop."

And that's when I came up with "eat what you like weight loss method". When I started to implement it, the weight finally began to come off.

It was that easy. I was done with dieting for good. I was also amazed at how the weight came off once I stopped depriving myself and started paring down my meals. Within a few months, I noticed my clothes were getting bigger and my self-confidence began to return.

Don't get me wrong, it took a good two years to shed that weight but once it came off, it *stayed* off. I had to trust that the weight would come off if I could stick to my new weight loss plan. And it worked. It's really not that big a deal.

The great thing was my skin wasn't stretched or saggy. More like I just got smaller and smaller all over. I lost it a little at a time just like I gained it a little at a time. The weight came off in increments, nothing drastic but slowly and, most importantly, *permanently.* All I did was cut down on my food. And that's what I continue to do now. I simply watch what I eat.

It was like it was staring me right in the face the entire time. And when you get right down to it, it's really just using your brain, isn't it? Don't overeat and you will lose weight. Duh. This was no miracle. This was common sense.

Why hadn't anyone ever told me this? Why did it take this much time—and effort and pain—for me to realize it? Why weren't the magazines and the media on to this already? Why? Because there's a billion dollar industry that doesn't want you skinny. They want you fat. If you lose weight, they lose business. And a lot of their business is from repeat customers.

Are you slapping yourself on the head yet? I was! Let me tell you one thing, I didn't think it could be that easy, but I had nothing to lose by trying it my way. So, I tried it. It worked! It worked like a charm. It took a while and I had to watch myself but I ate what I wanted. I didn't count calories and I didn't count carbs. I didn't carry some fat gram book around with me, either. All I did was cut my food intake back and eat most of my calories earlier in the day. That's all I did and it worked.

In review:
- ✓ Diets do not work and they cost you more than money in the long run.
- ✓ After I stopped dieting, I found an easier way to lose weight, calling it the "eat what you like weight loss method".
- ✓ I lost weight by gradually cutting back to just two light meals a day and one moderate/main meal. (Please not that when I say moderate meal, and I will throughout the book, I don't mean five or six sandwiches. I mean something *moderate* that tastes good and satisfies me but does not make me feel stuffed or bloated.)
- ✓ Breakfast and supper are my light meals.
- ✓ Lunch is my "eat what I like" meal.

Why you should Lose weight.

Reasons to lose weight:
- ✓ So you climb the stairs without wheezing.
- ✓ So you will look better.
- ✓ So you will feel better.
- ✓ Because you don't want to get sick with heart disease, diabetes or any of that other bad stuff.
- ✓ Because you're sick of being overweight.

You have to *want* to lose the weight.

One of the most important aspects to any weight loss strategy is the desire to lose the extra pounds. Without this, you're setting yourself up for failure.

In some ways, you have to take the "cruel to be kind" approach with yourself. You have to honest and admit that you're overeating. Wake up and get real. If you can't do this, you can't lose weight and no exercise or weight loss program is going to help you.

Do yourself a favor and write down everything you had to eat today, including drinks and snacks. Don't stop and *don't* fudge. No one is going to know you did this. It's time to face up to it. Look up the calories or the fat grams that might be in each of these food items.

Now that you've done it, are you surprised you consumed that much food? You probably are. I know I was. When I was overweight, I normally ate three big meals and at least two snacks *everyday*. This doesn't include the sodas I consumed either. I don't know why I thought I had to have all this food. I think I just got into a habit of overeating. And sometimes, that's all overeating is—a habit. If you can break the habit of overeating, you can lose the weight.

Looking back, I am embarrassed at myself. I made all kinds of excuse in order to "allow" myself to eat as often as I liked. One way I gave myself permission to snack was to tell myself that I was feeling weak: "I'm weak and tired. I better eat something! That candy bar looks great and will hit the spot!"

What do you tell yourself? What excuses do you make? Write them all down and be honest. Honesty is what's going to pull you through this. Admit you're playing games with yourself in order to make overeating okay. We get so upset when we find out that someone else has lied to us, but we readily lie to ourselves in order to justify what we do. However, this little game we play with ourselves is doing nothing but setting us up for failure.

Now, sit down and ask yourself this, "Why do I want to lose this weight?" And don't be arbitrary and said, "Because it would make me healthier." That's a given. Do you want to buy a bikini? Do you want to fit into the jeans you wore in high school? Whatever your real reasons are, admit them. There's nothing wrong with them. Maybe your reason is so you can keep up with your kids or hike the Appalachian Trail. It doesn't matter. What matters is that you want to do it.

I do know that most people who are overweight do not like being overweight. I didn't like it at all. If, however, you like being overweight and have "accepted" that you will always be this way, then good for you. But I don't think you would have picked up this book if you have accepted it. You don't have to accept it even if everyone else in the world says it's okay. It might be okay for them, but make your decision now if it's okay for you.

I have a friend, let's call her Jane. She's overweight and always complains about it. When I first started to lose weight, she would look at me with scorn and say, "You don't need to lose weight. *I* do."

A few times, I thought, "She's right," and I'd eat more than I should have. But then I realized she didn't want me to be thin if she wasn't. After that, I didn't let anything she said affect me. I was making a decision for myself, not for her and most certainly not for the rest of the world.

Other times, I would notice that people I work with would come up to me and said, "Look at how thin you're getting! You don't need to lose any more weight!" My mother even said it to me. But I did need to lose more weight because I hadn't reached my goal; in fact, I was only about twenty pounds into my plan when they started saying stuff like this to me.

People play games with themselves. Are you looking for an excuse *not* to lose weight? Ask yourself that and be completely honest. If you're looking for an excuse not to do it, you're not going to find it in this book. It's chock-full of hard truths. Some of those truths might sting a little but most of them should make complete sense—if you're willing to change your behavior.

However, if you are looking for an excuse not to lose the weight, you will find it. Maybe not here, but you can always talk yourself out of something if you try hard enough. Maybe you'll tell yourself that you don't have "time" to lose weight. You had "time" to overeat, didn't you?

You may also be playing the blame game. "If my husband would only…I'd lose the weight." Or, "No one cares if I lose the weight." Or, "It doesn't matter to anyone else if I do it, so why should I care?" I've even heard a close family member say, "I lost the weight once but nobody noticed so I just gained it all back."

If it all depends on someone else noticing your weight loss, then why bother? All this is is an excuse. It's an excuse to get back into lazy eating habits and an excuse to overindulge. It's a way to blame someone else while cocooning yourself in weight. It can't be your fault if others treat you like this, can it?

How about this? Blame it on yourself. You got yourself into this mess and only *you* can get yourself out of it. No one else is to blame. No one force-fed you or forced you to clean your plate or sneak that candy bar. You're playing a game with yourself here that has dire consequences. Overeating is a relief but it is only temporary. Right now it might not make you sick, but you better believe that on down the road, it will. Don't believe me? Why not ask your doctor what sort of maladies you can look forward to if you don't lose the weight?

Sure, this may sound harsh, but it's the truth. Being overweight does cause health problems. And the thing is, it's not that hard to lose it. It does take time and effort, but mostly all it takes is breaking a few bad habits like overeating.

How guilty do you feel after you finish eating? I know you feel guilt because I did. Once I started trying to lose weight and would eat a huge meal, I would just feel so disgusted with myself. I knew it was "bad" for me but I couldn't help myself. One day, I had a big lunch and then I had a big supper of a steak and French fries and a soda. For dessert, I had a brownie. I know I ate at least five-thousand calories that day. I was so overstuffed my belly was distending. Not only that, I felt on the verge of throwing up. I had eaten so much, my stomach couldn't contain it all and, quite disgusting, it was stuck in my throat.

That was torture and I vowed never to do it again.

How good would it be to never have to feel guilt again because you know that you can control your eating habits? I'll tell you how good it feels—it feels great! I've been there, believe me, and I know how it feels when you know you've eaten too much. It makes you feel awful. You feel disgust and repulsion for yourself. I did and I did because I knew I'd overeaten yet again and there was that more weight I'd have to try and lose later on. But I'd just push that thought away and not think about it.

Thinking like that is what caused me to gain the weight. It was only after I became honest with myself that I knew I could take control. And that's what this is all about—you taking control of your eating habits. It doesn't have to be intimidating and it's not that hard. Sure, this is a certain amount of sacrifice involved, but anything worth having is worth fighting for.

Aren't you tired of making excuses? Aren't you tired of not being able to climb the stairs without getting out of breath? Aren't you tired of staring at candy bars in the grocery store and not being able to say no?

Face up to *your* needs and make yourself a priority right here, right now. You are the most important person in the world to you. You are your own best friend. Start treating yourself as such.

In review:
- ✓ Admit to yourself that you want to lose weight.
- ✓ Write down everything that you eat and all of your excuses for snacking and overeating.
- ✓ Stop blaming others because you're overweight.
- ✓ Don't listen to other people who tell you you're fine "just the way you are." Ask yourself first if you feel fine with the way you are.
- ✓ Stop feeling guilty for being overweight. Take it upon yourself to do something about it, starting right now. Those feelings of guilt will soon be gone for good.

But So-and-So told me it was okay.

No one is going to *make* you lose weight. Some people might even tell you, "Why bother? Just accept yourself the way you are. It's okay."

Don't listen to these people. They are sabotaging you.

It's a hard truth to learn, but no one really wants you any skinnier, especially if they, themselves, are overweight. If you lose weight, they might have to take a closer look at themselves and do something, too. Be warned that if you do lose weight, you might make a few people angry.

A few years ago, I was at an in-service for my job and I noticed that a lady that works in another department had lost a bunch of weight. I went over to her and told her how great she looked and she smiled appreciatively. Later on, I asked the people at the table I was sitting at if they had noticed her weight loss. I couldn't believe what they said.

"Oh, she just looks awful," one of them said.

"Yeah," chirped in another one. "Her face is all drawn and she looks haggard."

"I didn't think she was *that* big to begin with," said another one.

I just stared at them. How rude! How insensitive! This woman had to have been over sixty pounds overweight and once she lost it, everyone lost the ability to be nice to her.

It's like they were saying: "She thinks she's *somebody* now! Look at the way she is! Always smiling and being happy! She's not like us anymore! How dare she?"

Want to know what I said in response to all that? I said, "Well, I think she looks much better and much healthier."

They did not appreciate my comment at all.

People told me I was fine just the way I was when I was overweight. "Oh, you're fine," they'd say. "Stop worrying." I never listened to them. I also knew that some of them were happy that I was overweight. It made *them* feel better about themselves. However, I didn't feel fine and I didn't like the way my body looked. I hid under big clothes and refused to take a look at myself in the mirror.

Instead of asking yourself what you have to gain by being thin, ask what you have to gain by being overweight. Are your friends overweight? What about your family members? Sure, we all know that overweight people don't want to hang out with skinny people. If this is what's holding you back, ask your pals if they'd rather you put your health at risk to be like them. This isn't high school and if you're still caving into peer pressure, you should ask yourself why. But more importantly, you should do what you want to do and *not let anyone else dictate your life for you.*

Being overweight is a very self-destructive behavior. People know it's not good for them and they know it's unhealthy. But if everyone else is doing it, why shouldn't they? I'll tell you why. It's not going to get you anywhere. It is going to make you sick and depressed. It might put you at risk for heart disease and diabetes. These are real risks.

My father has heart disease. He's overweight and has been since I can remember. He has to go into the hospital about once a year. He puts me and the rest of my family through a lot of worry because he refuses to eat less and exercise.

Believe me, you don't want to go through this and you do not want to put your family through it either. If you can do something to stop it, you should and not only for you but for your family. Because they do worry about you.

How overweight are you? Go to the scale right now and see. I know it's hard but you have to do it. Find the strength and step right up. How many pounds overweight are you? Let's say about forty. Now, go find something that is forty pounds and try to lift it. It's hard, isn't it? That's what your poor heart is doing everyday. It's lifting that extra forty pounds.

Can you imagine carrying around something that weighs forty pounds? Say for instance, a medium sized dog weighs about that much. You wouldn't want to carry Fido around all day, would you? But by having that extra weight on you, that's exactly what you are doing.

So why do most people refuse to face up to the fact that they're overweight? It's almost like some of them are rebelling, "You're not going to tell me what to do! I can do whatever I want to do and that means I can eat all I want!" You can't even say anything to overweight people now without them getting upset. And I don't. I know their pain because I went through it. When I see someone who's overweight, I want to hug them because anyone that is abusing their body in that way has something going on besides their love of food. When you make food the sole focus in your life, most of the time it's only masking some sort of pain or problem.

Ask yourself what it is. What do you fear most? Face up to it and then let it go. Get yourself back on track. Analyze your situation, keep a journal and detail your problems. Do whatever you have to do in order to face up to it. And once you do, you're going to be free. Food isn't going to matter that much anymore to you. It will be a way to fuel your body and nothing else. It won't have these overtones of happiness or feelings of elation once you look at it for what it is: Fuel for your body. Fuel so you can do the things you've always wanted to do. What other reason do you need?

In review:
- ✓ People will tell you it's okay to be overweight.
- ✓ It's okay to tell yourself that it's not okay.
- ✓ Weigh yourself today and face up to how overweight you are.
- ✓ Face up to any problems that may be holding you back.

I'll just have a taste.

Your brain is a fully functioning organ. It helps you make decisions and lets you know when to go to sleep. It's a great thing, your brain, but sometimes, you just don't use it, do you? And sometimes, it uses you.

Your brain might be what's messing with you and causing you to overeat and to snack. Maybe it's your emotions that cause this. And sometimes it's, "Ummm…that looks and smells so good!" Your brain recognizes food and suddenly, you're hungry, though you may have just eaten.

Many people overeat and snack because of their senses. If you smell something delicious, it's hard *not* to eat it. I know this to be very true. Whenever I pass a fast-food restaurant, my mouth waters and all I can think about is French fries and ketchup. Sometimes I give in. Most times, I do not.

And then there's this, "I'll just have a taste."

This may be one of the reasons you're overeating when you're really not hungry. Food today looks and smells so good. Just a bite here or there. No big deal. And it's really not a big deal. The big deal is that we don't stop at one bite. Most of us eat it all. Before we know it, it's all gone and in our bellies.

Learn to recognize these triggers. If you smell something delicious, take a big breath, smile and pass it by. You're going to eat later anyway, right? You don't need it right now even if it does look *so* good.

In review:
- ✓ One bite of one thing can lead to eating the whole thing. If you can cut out snacking altogether, you are ahead of the game from the get-go.
- ✓ Snacking, like overeating, is just a habit. It can be easily broken.

A perk.

One perk of cutting down on your meals is that you are going to save money.

I know this sounds ridiculous, but it's true. Just get a calculator and add up how much you'll save by not buying that candy bar or comfort food. You'll be surprised at how much it is.

The great thing about this is that you could take this extra money and put it towards your house payment and help pay it off early. Or you could save it for a vacation. You could spend it on new clothes. You could throw a party!

That should be incentive enough for just about anyone to stop overeating.

What we've covered so far.

Okay, let's review. I realized that diets weren't working for me. So, I decided that the best way for me to lose weight would be to stop dieting and start eating what I liked. However, I realized that I while I could eat what I liked, I couldn't eat it for every single meal. I could only eat it about once a day and still lose weight. Thusly, I began to implement the "eat what you like weight loss method".

For breakfast: I eat something small like a handful of nuts or a bowl of high fiber cereal or some fruit. It's just something small that tides me over till lunch.

For Lunch: I eat what I want, even if it's a cheeseburger and fries and soda. Also, I eat slowly and really enjoy my meal. After I'm done, I'm good to go and don't want anything else until supper.

For supper: Some days I just don't want that much to eat so I'll eat either a bowl of cereal or a bag of popcorn. Other days, I might have a chicken strip or two with some sort of veggie on the side or a salad. Whatever it is, it's a small amount of food. *My main meal for the day is over* and this is just something I eat to get me through the night.

I'm not saying what I eat is nutritionally sound and I do take a multi-vitamin as well as a calcium supplement. I'm not telling you to eat like me. I'm just telling you what *I* eat. What you put in your mouth is up to you. You can eat whatever you want for any of these meals—just eat a small breakfast, a moderate-sized lunch and a small supper. That way, your body is forced to catch up with itself and burn that fat.

And don't snack. Snacking might be the main culprit that's keeping you from losing weight. If you have to snack, have something small. Pickles or celery are good snacks and it's almost like you're not eating anything. Usually, when you get the urge to snack, all you're doing is maintaining a habit. So, if you eat something like celery or a pickle, you get that sensation but you're not overindulging. Eventually, you won't want to snack at all. Sounds crazy right now, but later on, you'll realize it's true.

The point is to *gradually* cut down on your food intake. You taught yourself to overeat and now all you're doing is teaching yourself how to cut back so you can get that weight off. Don't take it all away at once because then you're just setting yourself up for failure.

The point of this book is for you to find a way to do it for yourself. You can eat whatever you want, as I have said, but in smaller portions. You will realize that the less you eat, the less you will need. It's great. It really is. I couldn't believe what I used to eat and there is no way I could eat like that now. I believe one reason for this might be because my stomach shrank after I stopped overeating. It just can't hold what it used to. If I overeat now, I get so full that I feel ill.

It's as simple as that. And it worked for me.

If you want to try it another way, eat whatever you want at all meals. Go ahead and order up. Now once you're about half-way finished, stop. Push your plate away and wipe your mouth. Meal time is over. Whatever works for you is the best way. Just give it a try and see. What do you have to lose but that extra weight?

It's important to know that some days you will be hungrier than other days. That's fine. But on the days that you're not as hungry, don't force yourself to eat just because it's meal time. Eating when you're not hungry is just a habit, much like desserts and snacking.

In review:

- ✓ I eat something small for breakfast. Maybe just a piece of fruit or a handful of nuts or a bowl of high-fiber cereal.
- ✓ I have whatever I want for lunch and usually eat most of it.
- ✓ I don't snack. If you must snack, go for a gradual reduction and then try to cut it down to pickles or celery.
- ✓ If you want to eat three square meals a day, do so, but cut those three meals in half. *Only eat about half of each meal.*
- ✓ Drink plenty of water.
- ✓ It might be a good idea to take a multi-vitamin. Ask your doc.

An analogy.

One simple way to figure out how this works is to look at it like this. Say you have a dog and the dog is overweight. You decide that he needs to lose a little weight, so what do you do? You don't starve your dog, do you? No, you simply cut down his food. After you do this for a few weeks or months, he loses weight. It's that simple. Why wouldn't the same thing work for a person?

It does work for people. It's just that people want a miracle cure, a better way to do it, the easy-peasey way. And, in my opinion, this is *the* easiest way to do it. Cut down and the weight will come off.

"BUT I'M STARVING!"

Do you find yourself saying these words three, four or even five times a day? Are you really starving? More than likely, you're not. More than likely you do *not* have a tip on a famine but this little phrase might just be the reason you're overeating. We have this massive unfounded fear of starvation. It's time to face up to the reasons of why we have it and what we can do to get over it.

Let's begin by picking on diets again.

Diets initiate fear. When you say to yourself, "I'm going on a diet," you basically tell your body, "I'm going to start starving you." The body doesn't take kindly to this. "No," it says. "Please don't!" But you don't listen to it because you're overweight and you know you *have* to lose the weight. You don't care what you have to do! You are going to do it this time! This time for good and this new diet plan is going to work wonders.

Sometimes, it does work wonders. You do lose the weight while you're on this miracle cure. You can't believe it! You're so proud of yourself. However, as soon as you begin to eat normally again, the weight comes back and it comes back quick. Diets make people eat abnormally and once you go back to your normal routine, more than likely, you're going to gain the weight back.

Diets are not natural. They are not a natural way for you to eat. They are not a natural way for you to survive. This is why people usually gain the weight back.

The key is to gradually decrease your food intake until you are eating normally again and leaving yourself a little hungry at breakfast and at supper. This way is more manageable. You're not doing it all at once. This way is less intimidating. When you reach your weight goal, you will then eat enough to maintain your "ideal" weight, but not *extra* to put it back on. You will know your body's needs and will recognize when you're eating too much and know what to do to get back on track.

This is not dieting. This is changing your eating patterns. This is a gradual reduction of eating. Nothing more and nothing less.

Once you cut down on your food intake, it won't take anything to maintain it. You will only be eating enough to get you through the day. And you will be eating what you desire to eat.

It's important to know that your body was designed to handle famine. When we were hunting and gathering, there were long stretches of time when people didn't eat *anything*. We are genetically programmed to store fat. This ensures that we will get through those hard times when papa can't track down a wild animal.

The only problem with this is that there is NO FAMINE! But for some reason, people are afraid that all of the food is suddenly going to be taken away. *Eat what you can cause there's not going to be anymore. It's going to run out.*

Even before you begin a diet, you might say to yourself, "Better eat now because in a few days I'll be dieting." And guess what? Your body begins to store fat. There's not a

thing you can do about it, ei... After all, it's only doing
what it needs to do in order ... breathe. And it's only doing
what you told it to do. It's no... think, it's doing though that's
what it certainly seems like.

Why do people gain the weight back they've lost? I
think it's because they don't know what to do *after* they've
lost the weight. They're tired of dieting. It's time to resume
eating.

And who wouldn't be tired of dieting and/or
deprivation? It's hard to totally change your eating habits
and your taste buds. Who wants a rice cake when you can
have a chocolate chip cookie? You've been in deprivation
mode for so long, you're tired of it. You want a taste of
something good and you want lots of it to "make up" for all
that time you spent being miserable. You can't eat quickly
enough because you were, in fact, starving.

It's like you were a hibernating bear. You've slept for
the winter and now it's time to wake up and get back to
eating. In fact, it's like we're all in a hibernating bear mode.
Eat now because we'll be asleep all winter. But the bear
sleeps all winter and loses his weight. We don't.

It's a vicious cycle.

Diets make you miserable. Have you ever seen someone
on a diet that smiles and laughs all the time? No. Their faces
are drawn and they glare at you from across the restaurant.
They want what you're having but they *can't* have it.
They're on a diet. They wonder, "Why can't I eat like that
and still lose weight?" They don't know it, but they can!
They just can't overeat.

People love to eat food and there is nothing—
nothing!—wrong with eating. There is, however, something
wrong with overeating.

If you can get your head around the fact that you are not going to starve to death if you stop overeating, you will lose the weight. Overeating is nothing more than a habit. Just like drinking or smoking or gambling. It's a habit that takes over your life and becomes an addiction. It is an addiction that can be overcome. But you have to face up to it. And you, alone, have to do something about it.

So next time you're hungry, don't say, "I'm starving." Say, "I could eat a little." And then eat a little. Just switching those words around will help you so much it's unbelievable. Don't believe me? Try it and see for yourself.

In review:
✓ Diets are an unnatural way to eat.
✓ Overeating is a habit that *can* be broken.

Is it genetics?

Still not convinced? Well, let's tackle this issue of "It's genetics" with some common sense.

If you believe you're overweight because of genetics, do yourself a favor and find some family pictures from ten or twenty or thirty or even a hundred years ago. Go on now. Someone in your family has to have some pictures of your ancestors. My mother keeps ours. Now look closely at these people who have your genetics, who are in your bloodline. How many of those people are obese?

People were rarely overweight in the old days because there wasn't the abundance of food that we have nowadays so they *couldn't* overeat. They were also more active as most had vegetable gardens and few had cars. They had to walk a lot.

Also, keep in mind that overeating back then was not as readily accepted as it is today. Not only did they not have enough food, but they knew not to overeat. Life was just harder if you were heavy back then.

Another thing people do that I think is dangerous is to blame their weight on medical problems. By all means I do suggest you see a doctor. It really *is* a good idea. But if he/she tells you there's nothing wrong with you, don't be disappointed. Be happy that you're healthy! You can and will lose the weight by yourself.

Be sure to get checked for everything, from head to toe. Have your doctor check your thyroid and all of that stuff. If he finds something wrong, please follow his medical advice. It's time to get better isn't it? But we all know that more than likely, he won't find anything wrong. And let's get real here. To want something to be wrong with you that would explain the weight is just so sad. Why would you want to be sick? I know that weight problems are hard but you can take care of them without having to resort to desperate measures and that includes pretending there is something wrong with you medically.

I know this woman who is about four-hundred pounds. She always thought it was her thyroid that was keeping her from losing weight. It wasn't.

But the doctor agreed with her and she had it removed. Now she has to take pills everyday and the weight still hasn't budged. It's sad because she's a really nice person and I hate to see her go through that much pain. She couldn't face up to the fact that she was responsible for her weight gain and not her thyroid.

And then there is the old standby of gastric bypass surgery. This lovely operation entails a surgeon splitting open your belly and stapling your stomach so it's nice and small. If you overeat once you have this done, you'll get sick—physically sick. That is, if you make it through the operation without any complications.

This completely baffles me. People are mutilating their insides to lose weight. Stop and think about this. Do you know how complicated and dangerous this surgery is? I'll tell you: *VERY!* But people are lining up to do it.

Instead of having gastric bypass surgery, why not start today eating what you would if you had had it? You'll probably lose the same amount of weight without the hassle.

In fact, you *might* lose more. Pretend you had the surgery if you have to. If you have this surgery, you are going to have to worry about what you put in your mouth for the rest of your life. Why not start today?

If you are considering this surgery, it might be because you want it to fix your life. After you get it done, it is still up to you to fix it! It is up to you and you only to get this weight off. All you have to do is face up to the fact that you're overeating. You can do it on your own. You can save the money and the trouble! If you do my weight loss plan, you will lose the weight. Make my weight loss plan your alternative to gastric bypass! (By the way, your stomach will shrink *naturally* if you stop overeating as you won't be able to hold that much food anymore.)

I've know people who've gone to drastic measures, including getting their mouths wired shut. They literally pay someone to wire their mouth closed so they can't eat. And does it work? No. It won't work because people have to eat in order to survive. They just don't know when to stop.

We have scientists trying to find a "fat" gene. This is how preposterous it's gotten. Forget about cancer, we need to figure out the fat. Scientists a hundred years ago would have laughed if you told them to work on this project but now it's viable.

Would you cut off your pinkie finger to lose the weight? I know there are many people out there that will readily say yes to this and that makes me sad. Some might even give up both pinkies.

What drastic measures are you willing to take?

The thing is that you don't have to take drastic measures. All you have to do is to stop overeating. You don't have to stop eating, but you do have to stop *overeating.*

Sure, there may be emotional reasons behind overeating, but it can sometimes be a fear-based choice. My father is overweight because he grew up poor and they didn't have much food. Now he's making up for lost time because he has a fear of going back to that feeling of being hungry and helpless. He's treating himself to food now because when he was younger, he didn't receive any treats.

People have to stop treating themselves with food.

It's sad to say that we're doing all of this because we're not willing to cut back on food intake. We're mutilating ourselves and spending millions of dollars on research to explain it and the reason why is right in front of our faces. We eat too much! That's it, folks, that's the reason we're all overweight. Why do people have to have some *reason* for being overweight when all it boils down to the fact that they eat too much? Some people would rather mutilate themselves than to face up to the truth.

Why not do yourself a favor and stop overeating? That way, you won't have to go to these drastic measures. And, believe me, given the options, this is the easiest and least painful way to go about it.

In review:
- ✓ More than likely, it's not genetics that's keeping the weight on your body.
- ✓ See a doctor and get checked out from head to toe. He will let you know if something is amiss.
- ✓ Drastic measures like gastric bypass surgery to lose weight are dangerous.
- ✓ Make my weight loss plan your alternative to gastric bypass surgery. Try to eat what you would have if you had *had* the surgery.

A little insight.

Do you know babies refuse to eat when they're not hungry? You can try to make them take a bottle but they will shake their little heads and scrunch up their noses. They don't want anymore! *Wah!* It's true. So why are you doing it to yourself? If you're not hungry, just don't eat. Go find something fun to do, even if it's just playing with your kids. They love you bunches. If you don't have kids, play with…well, do something besides eating.

Remember, it's a habit. Break the habit!

Another good thing that will help you is to think of how a baby is on a feeding schedule. They usually get hungry at about the same times. If you schedule your meals to fall at about the same time every day, you will get on a schedule and this will help you lose weight.

Super-size!

It is never a good idea to super-size your meal. If you do nothing else at least stop doing this. Those extra calories are just going to sit on your body somewhere.

If you are at a fast-food restaurant and they ask if you would like to super-size, tell them, "No, thanks." I mean, you're already having fast-food. You don't need anything extra. If you buy extra, you'll feel *obligated to eat extra.*

But that fast-food restaurant wants you to feel like you're getting a little extra food for a little extra money. They're making money and you're making yourself gain weight. And you think you're getting a bargain!

So, whenever they ask, just take a moment and ask yourself, "Why would I do that?" You do it because we are all being programmed to overeat in order to fill the pockets of these gigantic corporations. They super-size your meal, you super-size their bank accounts, the food super-sizes your pants. The way I see it, they already have enough money.

Another thing. Restaurants always want us to get our money's worth, don't they? So, when you order a meal, it's usually enough to feed two (and sometimes more) people. Why not share a meal? My husband and I sometimes order one dish and then split it. We had gotten out of the habit of doing this when we recently visited a pancake house. They brought me an omelet that was the size of my arm! It was enough to feed an army. And the thing was, I felt bad because I didn't get to eat it all. If you share a dish, then there's less chance of any leftovers and that means less guilt.

Another thing, I never order appetizers and rarely order drinks at a restaurant. I just go for the main course. Sometimes, if you're really hungry, you'll want an appetizer, but just know that your waitress will soon bring your food and then you can eat until you're satisfied. Yes, you can wait.

One last thing. If you can get into the habit of ordering water whenever you're dining out, go for it. The amount of calories in sodas is astronomical. Think of all the weight you could lose if you cut them out.

In review:

✓ Never, ever super-size.

✓ Share a meal at a restaurant. (This doesn't mean you're cheap. Don't be embarrassed to do it, either. Just ask for an extra plate.)

✓ Forget appetizers. They cost way too much and you don't need them anyway. Your food will arrive shortly. If you have to chew something, chew a piece of gum while you wait.

✓ It's a good idea to drink water instead of sodas when dining out.

Skinny people don't suck.

"Skinny people suck!" This girl I know said this once and instead of looking at her like she was crazy, I felt pity for her. She was overweight and she just wouldn't face it. Know what else she was doing? She was blaming everyone else for her weight problems and she was taking it out on skinny people. Skinny people were her enemies! She hated them!

We're so obsessed with weight—and, again, we could blame it on the media and those skinny models!—but the thing is, being overweight isn't good for your health. Blaming all the skinny people is just a way to deflect the responsibility. I know that's what I was doing anyway.

Many overweight people I know take the martyr approach to it. They hate anyone who tries to tell them how much better they will feel once the weight comes off. They even get upset at their doctors! But they know deep-down that they need to lose the weight, otherwise skinny people wouldn't upset them so much.

It's natural to feel envy for all those super-skinny people. I know sometimes I look at a model in a magazine and the old green-eyed monster comes out. So I think, *If I stopped eating all-together, I could look like that.*

But I'm not going to stop eating all-together. I like to eat. Going out for a meal is one of my favorite things to do. I'm not stopping because of some super-skinny girl in a magazine.

But I do *control* it. I don't eat and eat until my cheeks are bursting and my belly is distending. I take my time and eat slow and devour the delectable taste of my food, even if I'm just eating a bowl of cereal.

Have you heard the myth about how skinny people have a higher metabolism than overweight people? Who made this up? No, I don't think they do and until medical science proves me wrong, I'm sticking with my opinion. Sure, everyone claims to know that one person who can eat anything they want and never gain an ounce. I believe this type of person is an urban legend. I don't know anyone like that. If I did, I'd put them in an eating contest.

I think that people are just not watching how skinny people eat. People say this about me because I eat what I want. They just don't notice that I'm not eating the whole thing.

Some people do have faster metabolisms—it's just that it's not *that* much faster. These people are human and the same rules of eating still apply.

Find someone whom you believe to be this type of person. Watch them closely. Exactly what are they eating? Usually, they're not eating everything in sight; in fact, most of these people I know eat like rabbits. Some of them eat several little meals day. Some of them eat a big meal once a day and that's it, no breakfast and no lunch. Some of them just don't eat that much at all. That's why they're so skinny! It usually has nothing to do with metabolism.

It could also be that they're anorexic. If so, they've got bigger problems than you or me and we shouldn't put them down for it. We should offer our support to them. They need it.

I've had people ask me why I can eat whatever I want and not gain weight. I tell them that I don't overeat, that's how. They don't believe me. One person in particular did this to me, so I invited her to lunch one day. She couldn't believe what she witnessed. We went to a buffet and after I had a small salad, I got a plate of mashed potatoes and gravy, roast beef and some veggies. I ate what I wanted off the plate, leaving it about half-full, then I got a little macaroni and cheese and a chicken strip. Then I had a piece of pie for dessert. All while sipping on sweet tea.

She was beside herself. "How do you do that?"

I told her, "I can do it because I probably won't eat much more for the rest of the day. *That's* how I do it."

"Wow," she said and finally got it.

Isn't it time to stop worrying about what everyone else is doing to stay so thin? Find *your* method and stick to it.

In review:

✓ Skinny people have their own problems, so leave them alone.

✓ Skinny people stay skinny by not overeating. They know when to cut back.

✓ Eat what you want and stop when you're satisfied.

#1 Rule to lose weight: Stop overeating!

If you stop overeating, you will lose weight. It might not come off all at once, like some of those "miracle" pills and diets promise you, but it will come off.

You need to realize that nothing happens overnight. There are no overnight successes in anything and that includes losing weight. Take time to do it. Be patient. Sure, people may lose weight faster than you. But just watch as they gain it all back. Meanwhile, you will continue to lose and you won't be driving yourself crazy in the process.

Misconceptions about diet sodas and other myths.

Diet sodas are calorie-free and help you lose weight. While it's true that they are low in calories, this, in my opinion, is a *huge* misconception.

Have you ever noticed that people who drink diet sodas are rarely thin? The only skinny people I've seen drink the stuff were on the commercials for them.

Usually, diet sodas are a symptom of being overweight rather than a cure. Many—not all—but many people who drink them were already overweight before they started. Also, since they're volume eaters, i.e. people who eat enormous meals for every meal and snack, they think that they can drink/consume more if it's called low calorie.

So, it's not doing you that much good to drink it, is it? If you can wean yourself off of it and just drink water, you are going to see a big improvement. (You also won't have all those chemicals in your body.) If you have to have soda, why not just try the regular kind for a week or so and see if you see any improvement?

This also applies to food. I know this couple who are obese. They are always trying to cut back and lose weight. One day, I was at their house and they had, of all things, diet donuts. Diet donuts! That's an oxymoron! Those two words do not go together but they ate 'em all up in one sitting because they were "diet".

While we're at it, let's touch on those non-fat food products. I heard somewhere that these items usually have more sugar and more sugar has more calories and that's going to get you nowhere. It sounds like a good idea, though: "Only a hundred calories!" Or "Low Fat!" We take this to mean that we can eat as much of these foods as we like. We can't. And the reason we can't is because the manufacturers of these "low fat" foods normally substitute sugar for fat. That's a lot more calories your body has to burn.

Have you ever tasted these low fat creations? They taste like cardboard. So, why waste time, money and calories on something you really don't even like? Just eat what you like, but don't overdo it.

In review:
- ✓ Diet sodas don't really seem to work that well.
- ✓ It might be a good idea for you to cut them out all together.
- ✓ Instead of drinking diet sodas, maybe you could switch to juice or water.
- ✓ Other "diet" foods should be handled with caution as well. Don't buy into the "low fat" mythology.

Guzzling.

Used to be, you could stop at a convenience store and grab a soda in a paper cup. Now they don't have paper cups. They have vats. From thirty-two ounces to forty-four and I've even seen eight-six ounces of soda. Huge drinks in astronomical sizes—all under two bucks.

Sure, it sounds cheap enough. Two bucks really isn't that much. But if you're drinking gallons of soda a day, you're paying a much, much higher price. Think of all the calories in those sodas that add up to extra pounds. Think of all the blood, sweat and tears you're going to spend trying to get those extra pounds off. Is it worth it for a bargain? No, it's not.

So, if you find yourself going for the vats of soda, *stop.* Don't guzzle them. If you can do this, you will lose weight. If you want something to drink, pick up a small fruit or vegetable juice or a bottle of water instead.

You will notice that as you pare down what you're eating, you will become more aware of how many calories you're consuming. And if you waste calories, you'll want it to be on something a lot more exciting than a vat of soda.

In review:
✓ Don't buy vats of convenience store soda.
✓ Go for a fruit or vegetable juice or water instead.

You are not a big, fat pig!

When eating, don't say to yourself, "I am such a big, fat pig! I shouldn't be eating this!" You have to eat to survive. Just say, "Oh, this tastes good but I'm going to stop when I'm satisfied." And here's the trick: *Stop when you're satisfied.*

Don't hate your body. You're not getting another one, you know? This is it. Pledge to make it the best body you can get.

Figure out your relationship with food. Eat only when you are hungry and stop eating in the middle of the meal for a couple of minutes. This allows you time to see if you're getting satisfied. If you can't hold much more food without feeling sick, then it's time to stop.

If you eat regular meals about the same time everyday, your body will automatically adjust to these times and let you know when it's hungry. And when it gets hungry, you will get a little burn going on in your belly and it will growl. When you're eating, it's also a good idea to just sip whatever drink you're having. In Europe, most people do this. (Many of them only drink water with their meals.) They eat and *then* they drink. Remember, your food already has some water in it, so you're not going to get parched while you eat.

Another thing to do is to eat slowly. Taste your food. Do the Gomer Pyle rule of "Twenty-five chews!" If you take time to taste your food by chewing it thoroughly, your meal will be that much more satisfying. I know people who inhale food. That's right, they don't eat it, they inhale it. I can't even imagine how they even taste it. And the kicker is that they eat so fast they don't even realize they're full! This makes them eat more than they need.

Your body will thank you for it and, I hate to be gross, but you'll get a lot less gas. If you eat fast, you also swallow air which leads to…you know.

In review:

- ✓ Stop calling yourself names and don't hate your body.
- ✓ Eat only when hungry and eat regular meals at around the same time if possible. Eat these meals slowly and chew food.
- ✓ Sip drinks instead of guzzling them when you eat.

But there are children starving in China!

People, let's face facts here. We are not in China and, thank God, because I don't dig that whole communist thing.

When eating, don't worry about cleaning your plate and don't worry about the starving children in China. (Sorry, kids.) Sure, the day might come when the gravy train is no more, but let's not worry about that until it happens, okay?

Another thing, when you're at someone's house (i.e. relatives) and they want you to eat and you don't want to, take a bite but refuse the rest. If they get upset, they need to get a life.

If you really want to be a nice person, save all that money you'll have from not overeating and send it to those starving children in China. They have all kinds of charities that help these poor kids out. You help them gain weight, they help you lose it. How nice is that?

In review:
- ✓ If you are worried about the starving children in China (or elsewhere) find a reputable charity and send them some money for food. Don't try to eat *for them.*

Overeating—sometimes, it will happen.

Whenever I travel, I tend to overeat. I readily admit that. I can't get enough of local flavor and I look forward to eating all kinds of new things.

When this happens, all I have to do is compensate after I return from my trip by not eating as much as I did the previous week. That simply means I have to cut back when I return from vacation.

If you do overeat, don't beat yourself up. You can and will do better next time! Just cut back on a few of your other meals and the extra pounds will come off. You just have to give your body a little nudge. Remember, if you overeat, you will not be that hungry later. Just listen to your body and start eating when you finally become hungry again.

In review:
- ✓ Know that sometimes, you will overeat.
- ✓ After it happens, just cut back again and it shouldn't be that big of a deal.

Curing your sweet tooth.

Chocolate cake does not love you. It will make you gain weight. But, you do need to eat a piece every now and again.

What? Yeah, you heard me.

If you deprive yourself all the time, you are only going to binge later on. Deprivation is like you're saying to yourself, "Once I start dieting, I can't eat sweets ever again." Yes, you can! You just can't eat them all the time.

When I first starting losing weight, I had a sweet tooth the size of Caesar's Palace. I had to have my chocolate! At first I had a hard time reconciling this, but I finally figured it out. I could eat something sweet but only in small quantities. Solution? I bought a bag of snack-sized candy bars and I ate one a day after I ate supper. After a few months of this, I didn't even want it once a day, maybe every other day and so on and so forth until I didn't want it at all. I began to notice that I was throwing old candy bars in the garbage because they weren't being eaten. That was money well wasted.

If you want a cookie, eat a cookie—just don't eat the whole bag. Let me rephrase that: Eat *only* one cookie. Save some for tomorrow or for the day after tomorrow or for next week.

Soon, maybe you won't feel like eating a cookie. When you start cutting them out you will find that you don't want them as often. It may take another month before you crave one. Once you crave it, go get it. But only that one time. Stop after you've finished and promise yourself that you can have another one soon, just not right now.

It may be hard to believe, but once you start this behavior, your sweet tooth will diminish along with your dress size. You won't crave sweets like you used to.

The key here is to *not* deprive yourself. You need to learn to limit your intake of these delicious foods and enjoy them in moderation. You can have your cake and eat it, too. You just can't eat it *every single day.* And the kicker? You probably won't even want it every single day.

If you can get into the habit of bypassing the cookie aisle in the grocery store, it won't be long until you stop thinking about it altogether. I don't. I have to pass it to get to the other aisles, but it never catches my eye.

If you can't cut down to once a week, do this: Cut down to once a day. Some of you may have a bigger sweet tooth than others so you may have to start out slow. You have to start somewhere and if you give everything up all at once, you will be right back to where you started. This is a proven fact and this is why drastic deprivation diets normally don't work.

Remember, what you're going for is a gradual reduction in your food, including sweets. Cut down a little a day, day by day. Yes, it is going to take longer to lose weight when you do this. Yes, it might be a whole year before you get all your weight off, maybe even two, maybe even three. But most of us can't do it all at once and if we try, we are only setting ourselves up for failure. And once you fail at weight loss, it's hard to get back on the bandwagon, isn't it? There are no quick fixes. You are going for a life changing pattern here.

In review:

✓ Just like it took time to put the weight on in the first place, it will take time to get it off.

✓ If you want a cookie, have a cookie but wait a few days before you have *another.*

✓ Never deprive yourself.

My addiction.

I readily admit that I am addicted to soda pop. I have to have one when I get up in the morning. I drink it instead of coffee, which I don't like. Sometimes, I have it with lunch, too. I figure if I stopped drinking soda all-together, I would probably lose five pounds without even trying.

But I can't. Or rather, I won't.

Since I don't want to give it up, I decided that I could have my soda and drink it, too. It's my vice. I think everyone needs at least one vice. Without having one, how boring would life be?

Most times, I don't even drink the whole can. Maybe just half and sometimes all I want is a sip.

Maybe you don't like soda but you like brownies. Why not have a special treat of a brownie a few times a week? Pick your poison and let that be your special treat. You don't have to overindulge and you can switch it around to something different if you like. And it gives you something to look forward to. "I get my brownie at lunch today!" Soon, you'll just want a bite or two of it and eventually, you might not want it at all.

It's up to you. But by cutting out everything you enjoy, you do nothing but suck the joy out of life and that's no fun, is it?

In review:

✓ Pick something that you like to eat and indulge yourself a few times a week. This helps to keep the fun in life and you don't feel deprived.

Food: It's everywhere!

We are being encouraged to overeat. Food, food, food! It's everywhere! It's on the TV, on the billboards, in the magazines, in the newspapers. It's inside of nice restaurants that advertise their delicious products so well *no* one can resist. No matter what we do, we are besieged with advertisements for food throughout the day. And during the night, we are bombarded by infomercials to help us lose the weight that the food companies wanted us to gain.

No wonder we are so overweight.

Need to run an errand? On your way there, you pass the ice cream parlor and they just got a new flavor. *Mmm...ice cream.*

Sitting back and reading the newspaper? Wow, more food all over the place and recipes galore! Come to think of it, I might just be a little hungry after all.

Ready to watch your favorite TV show? How's about a little popcorn to go along with the sitcom antics? Sure, and a soda too. Oh, look, there's a commercial for that new pie and I would love to have a piece of that. I'll have to pick that up next time I'm at the grocery store.

Do you see what's going on here? The people who make these oh-so-delicious foods just want your money. That's why they advertise the pizzas and the chocolate cakes and all that good stuff. They know that they make your mouth water in anticipation. They're smart and they're getting rich off of us.

My advice? During commercials, put the TV on mute or get up and do a few small tasks like balancing the checkbook or folding a load of laundry. But don't sit there and watch that parade of food. It's like putting a steak in front of your dog and expecting him not to eat it. It won't happen. You are triggered by commercials to want what you don't have. It's subliminal. It's making all of us gain weight.

We are close to food at all times. It's on TV and on the radio. This makes it stay on our minds. It seems like we would get sick of food because we are surrounded by it so much. However, this is just not the case. I think the reason why is because we need food in order to survive, so we'll never get sick of it.

The food industry knows this. There is this gigantic industry prospering because we're all overeating. While they're tooling around in fancy cars and jetting off to exotic islands, the rest of us are paying the price. And we're paying the price because we can't resist the urge to overindulge. And that's really all we're doing when we're overeating. We're overindulging. A little overindulgence isn't necessarily a bad thing; it's okay occasionally. We have to find a way to stop doing it all the time.

We're also always told not to "deprive" ourselves. It is this mindset that has us all buying bigger and bigger clothes. It needs to stop. It has to stop sometime. People have to wake up. A revolution should be born.

If all of us woke up and took it upon ourselves to stop overeating, the dieting industry would collapse. There wouldn't be a need for new fad diets or, thank God, infomercials. No new "miracle" pills would be developed and these people would have to get real jobs.

I was once watching a documentary which featured some old news footage on TV and my husband sat up in his seat and said, "Would you look at those people? None of them are overweight."

I stared at the TV. He was right. The reel was about twenty-five years old and none of the people were overweight. They were average, everyday people. In today's world they would have been considered skinny. *That was only twenty-five years ago.*

How did they do it back then? They didn't overeat, that's how. In that amount of time, this epidemic has taken over our lives. We are consumed with food and with eating and also with shedding it through dieting. But how did we get here?

It's very simple when you get right down to it. Advertising triggers us to indulge ourselves. That makes us eat more than we should. Then, we need something to help us lose the weight. This makes us go on diets. We're constantly reminded of food and then we're constantly reminded that we have to lose weight.

But that's not where it stops.

Once you're overweight, you need medical attention but not only that, you will also need drugs. So you go to the doctor and he gives you a pill which helps you to live. This helps the pharmaceutical companies stay in business. And, boy, do they ever want to stay in business because that business is Big Business, with a capital "B". There are all kinds of pills for high blood pressure and cholesterol. If you're overeating because you're depressed, here's a pill for that too! The drug companies are racking up. There's a pill for everything! They can fix just about anything with a little pill.

They are turning us into a nation of druggies.

How sad is this vicious cycle? We're not just saying yes to food, we're saying yes to the way of life the advertisers are giving us. We're saying yes to the drug companies that are going make us feel "better". All of us want to eat the best foods, go on the best diets, see the best doctors and take the best drugs. And advertisers make sure we do. Sure, if you have high cholesterol, you probably do need a pill. So, why not do something now so you don't have to take a pill? Why not make the decision for yourself that this is your life and you would like to live it without being overweight or dependent on drugs?

In the end, we are being played by advertisers. They are advertising better drugs and better foods and better diets. They are doing it for big corporations who are prospering off of our health problems and our food addictions. They are making money off our inability to control ourselves. They make us want what we really don't need. And that we could easily do without. It's up to you to ignore their messages. If you make an effort to do this, advertisements won't affect you that much. And that will help you lose weight, too.

In review:
- ✓ Food is everywhere and it's hard to escape.
- ✓ Learn to tune out triggers such as advertisements.
- ✓ Take a stand today to do something about your weight so you do not have to depend on drugs later on.

The Latest diet craze.

Now you're sitting at home watching TV and you see an advertisement for the latest diet craze. The image you see is of super-skinny people who are just grinning and having the time of their lives. Sometimes they're at the ocean and sometimes they're hiking and sometimes they're smiling at their children. They are the happiest they have ever been. And it's all because they used *this* particular diet plan which is so quick and easy you won't believe the results!

They're right. I don't believe them. And that's because I've tried most of their diets and none of them have ever worked. But, I will readily admit that when I see some of these commercials, I do get tempted: "That last five would come off in no time!" Sometimes I even go as far as to watch for the commercial again and again just so I can analyze it.

But then I regain my senses and stop myself. I don't need to spend money on this junk. I can do it myself. But it is so easy to get tempted into that "lose weight quick" way of thinking they portray on the TV.

Aren't you tempted?

You shouldn't be. However, you usually are because when you see the perfect diet on TV or read about it a magazine, it looks so easy. I can do this one. I *have* to do it. I don't care how much it costs. This is the one for me. The more you see of these images, the more it settles in your mind. Lose weight! It only takes two weeks! Blah, blah, blah.

You start thinking, "Hey, that's a neat way to lose weight. I'm going to try that. It can't be *that* bad." It's probably not that bad. But if you don't plan on staying on it for the rest of your life, it's not going to keep your weight down.

If you didn't know diets existed, would you go on one? No, you would naturally cut back by curbing your appetite. But we've confused our bodies so much they don't know what to do anymore. By constantly overfeeding ourselves, we have entered into a vicious cycle of weight gain.

It's important to realize that these companies get a lot of their profits through repeat business. I don't think it's a conspiracy and they're really not doing it on purpose. But they do know that you want to lose weight and you're willing to try about anything. So, why not try to not overeat? If nothing else, it's a lot cheaper. In fact, it's the only diet plan where you'll actually *save* money.

In review:
- ✓ Most diets do not work.
- ✓ Learn to ignore "miracle" diets advertised on TV and in magazines.
- ✓ Lose the weight yourself and save some money.

Is it worth it?

A second on the lips, equals forever on the hips. Someone once told me that and it is so true. Before you start to overeat, ask yourself if that one bite is worth all the work you're going to have to put in to get rid of it.

It's usually not. You know it and I know it so let's stop it right now.

Tips.

Here are just a few tips to help you in your quest to lose weight.

- ✓ *Eat a variety of stuff* that you like and crave. If you do this, you're not depriving yourself. Just eat small amounts.
- ✓ *Don't deprive yourself of food*—EVER! This is how that silly little battle between you and the candy bar got started in the first place. Recognize this and move on with your life.
- ✓ *Only eat when you are hungry*—physically hungry. Listen and feel for the signs of hunger like your belly growling. If you're not getting any signs, don't eat!
- ✓ *Stop giving food so much power over your life.* Stop scheduling your life around it. Sometimes, you will miss a meal here or there and that's just life.
- ✓ *Do not eat in front of the TV* or while you're reading or while doing anything else. Eat at a table and enjoy every single bite.
- ✓ *Eat slowly!*
- ✓ *Realize that when you're done eating, it won't be long until you eat again*, so don't worry if you throw half of your sandwich away.
- ✓ *Stop worrying about the starving children in China.* Send them some money instead.

- ✓ *The fear of being hungry is what most people are afraid of.* Why? Do you think that you will never eat again? That's just illogical.
- ✓ *You will have to watch how much you eat for the rest of your life.* Not what you eat but *how* much. It takes time to get to this point. Give yourself time. Don't try to cut down on everything the first day. Gradually build up to it. If you have to start with three full meals, do that, but don't snack and *don't* eat at night.
- ✓ *Do not—do not!—start out by skipping meals.* Or by cutting everything out. Do not think that you can do this more quickly by starving yourself. You are changing your eating habits over a period of time, not overnight.
- ✓ *It takes time to lose weight*, just like it took time to gain weight. There are no microwave-quick solutions here.
- ✓ *Ask yourself if you're afraid to lose the weight.* What are you afraid of? Starvation? Loneliness? Figure out what it is and move on.
- ✓ *Some days, you will overeat* and some days you won't overeat. This doesn't mean you're going to waste away. It means your body has to catch up with itself.
- ✓ *What I am telling you is not a revolution.* It is common sense. The diet industry doesn't want you to use your common sense because if you did, you wouldn't need their products.
- ✓ *If you're feeling faint or lightheaded, it's probably not due to lack of food.* If you've eaten your meals, you should be fine. If you do feel weak, you might want to see the doctor. (As I have said, it is a good

idea to get your doctor's opinion before you start any weight loss plan and that includes this one.)

✓ *At night, your belly will growl. You will be hungry.* Make it to the next day and once you start this pattern, your body will only get hungry when it's meal time. Just like a baby is on an eating schedule, so should you be.

✓ *If it's not in your kitchen cabinet, you can't eat it.* Just try it one time. Bypass the cookie aisle in the grocery store just once. Don't buy a candy bar at the convenience store just once. If you are obsessing about a cookie or a candy bar, promise yourself that you can have it tomorrow. By the next day you will, more than likely, feel foolish and not want it.

✓ *If you gain a little weight at first, don't beat yourself up.* Just start a new day, everyday.

Food obsession.

I think we all obsess about food. When are we going to eat again? Where are we going to eat? And, most importantly, what are we going to eat?

Food, food, food.

It rules our lives. In some cases, it takes *over* our lives. I know it took over mine. Mealtimes were most important to me and what I looked forward to. I based my whole day around them, in fact.

The thing to remember is to not let food take over your life. Food does become as much as an obsession as overeating becomes a habit. If you can divert your attention away from it, you can get your cravings under control.

If you find yourself roaming into the kitchen after you've already eaten supper, roam right back out. Set a time limit. "I won't go in there for one hour." If the hour passes and you still want something to eat, you need to realize that this is how you gained weight in the first place. Are you going to let it beat you again?

Even today, after all my struggles to lose weight, I still sometimes find myself going into the kitchen and shoving crackers in my mouth. Sure, I might be a little hungry, but I'm not wasting away. Most times when I do this, I am either bored or it's a diversion from a job I need to do around the house. I don't need those calories. I'm just eating to be eating.

Are you eating for distraction? If so, it's time to stop. Are you eating because you're bored and there's nothing else to do? Find something else. Read a book or go for a walk, do whatever you have to do to stop. I do believe that sometimes people are just looking for something to occupy their minds and food fits the bill.

If you are eating a moderate meal at least once a day, and eating two smaller meals along with that, you shouldn't have to eat anymore until the next day because your body has stored up those calories to use up later. Now, if you continue to eat after this, that just means there will be more calories to burn. *Give your body a chance to catch up with itself.*

Your body is just doing its job when it packs on the pounds. That's what it's programmed to do. When we were hunting and gathering, this helped us survive through the winter when there wasn't as much food around. Here's a newsflash, folks: We're not hunting and gathering anymore. But some of us still think we are. Sure, if something happens, overweight people will survive longer. But in the meanwhile, they will probably have more health problems.

You need to know that once you start losing weight, your stomach will grumble. You will feel hunger pangs. Don't take this as a sign to fill up. Don't rush for a pack of donuts. Feeling hungry is natural and when you get a hunger pang, know that your body is using up some of that extra fat it has stored. This is a good thing. It means you're losing weight!

Don't undermine it by having a silly thought of passing out or of being weak. If you feel weak all the time when you start this, go see a doctor. But most times, you're feeling weak because you are psyching yourself out.

Before you put that cookie or whatever in your mouth, please do yourself a favor and ask yourself this: *Am I eating because I am truly hungry or is it because I'm bored? Or is something bothering me?*

When we go through hard times, we use food as a way to comfort us. I know when I am stressed, I want to eat everything in sight. And the trick is to realize what you're doing and put a stop to it.

Once you face up to what's bothering you, your obsession for food will wane. Facing fears of the unknown—or the known, for that matter—is something that won't only help you lose weight but it will also help you with everything in life. This pain and suffering, which is mostly self-induced, will be gone once you do this.

That's all overeating is. It's self-inflicted pain. You're not overeating because you think you'll die from starvation. Maybe you're overeating because you're worried about something. Usually, those types of worries are unfounded and are only in your head to distract you from doing something else. Maybe you didn't get a promotion. Maybe you're concerned with someone's health. Maybe your kids are driving you crazy. Sit down, take a minute and ask yourself what it is that you fear most. Let it come to you. Figure it out, face it and move on.

Another reason we overeat is because we are so stressed with all that we have to do. Take out some of the things in your life that are causing you stress. You can't do it all. No one can. Just like you can't have it all, just like you can't eat everything you want without gaining a bunch of weight.

Eating is a pleasurable act. Everyone loves good food. I know I do. I'm not afraid to admit it and you shouldn't be either. But when you become obsessed with it and with mealtimes, I believe you're only distracting yourself from something. Mine was that my life wasn't working out how I thought it would it. Once I faced up to that, everything fell into place. Once you do, the same thing should happen for you.

I do know that most people who are overweight don't like being overweight. Many people who need to lose weight may not be able to do so because of some block. Search out your block and confront it head on. Smash that block to bits. That block is what is keeping you from leading a fuller, healthier life. It needs to be destroyed.

In review:
✓ Food obsession may be a just a diversion from life.
✓ It may also be boredom relief.
✓ Find out what triggers your snacking and/or overeating.

Mind control.

It's all about mind control. (Oh, it's getting creepy!) You think, "I'm hungry," when you're really not and the urge to binge/snack/overeat comes on strong and you give in to it. STOP! When was the last time you ate? Ten minutes ago? You're not hungry. You're *BORED!*

Food is just food and all it is a way to fuel your body. That's it. Get the emotional stuff out of your system and lose that weight.

Binge eaters.

Keep in mind, that you are changing your life—not just the size of your clothes. In order to keep the weight off, you will have to change. There is no way around this. Ask yourself if it's worth it. It *should* be worth it. You want to be healthy and lead a good life free from calorie counting and bingeing.

Know you will be frustrated. Know that sometimes you will binge and sometimes you will overeat. The key is that when this happens, don't go back to what you were doing before. Start a new day, everyday. Forgive yourself if you overeat. Tell yourself that you will do better tomorrow and then *do better tomorrow*. This is mostly self-control and discipline and willpower. Eventually, it will become a habit. It will also build your self-esteem and willpower. Willpower is a big thing here. Tap into your willpower and you will be unstoppable. You have to create new good habits in order to destroy the old bad ones.

Food shouldn't dictate our behavior, but we let it. If you have a food obsession, it will take over your life and will leave you feeling helpless and hopeless over a binge. There is nothing worse than staring at an empty bag of potato chips and knowing that you ate the whole thing. I've done it and I'm sure you've done it, too.

Stress can make the best of us binge. I've been upset about something and then I'll find myself in the kitchen shoving food into my mouth. Sometimes I do it because I'm bored. Whatever your reason is, just know you can stop it. And you stop it by simply refusing to do it in the first place. Stop it one time and the next time will be that much easier. All you have to say is, "I am not doing this."

Learn to recognize the signs of a binge. Accept that you are doing it and take a deep breath, get a piece of paper and a pen and sit down at the table. Now write out whatever comes to your mind and how you're feeing. It might go a little something like this: "I'm fat and ugly and no one loves me and I don't love myself and I am so confused and hurt and angry I can't control my eating! Why can't I control my eating?! I hate my food addiction and I hate myself and I hate everything in the world right now and I just don't know why I do this to myself. It's crazy! I am only punishing myself and I know it! It's too hard to quit! It's too hard to stop. I can't stop. I just can't stop right now."

Cry, spit, and fume. Scream at the top of your lungs if you have to. Do anything to redirect your anger from bingeing. Stomp around and get good and angry. Let all that hot air out. Let all that frustration and name calling of yourself go away. Send everyone out of the house for a day so you can have some privacy. Take as long as you need to deal with your feelings. Face up to them. You have to get this out! So get it out now. If you're frustrated at your significant other, write it down. Write down what you're frustrated at and then write down how it makes you feel.

If you can do this, then you have redirected yourself from binging. Now, all the things you have written down aren't true, of course, but that's what you're feeling right at that moment. Don't censor yourself one bit. Cry if you have to. It's good to cry and get all that frustration out of your system. Get it all out and know you will feel much better once it is gone. Once you write it down, you'll see just how ridiculous it is.

When you are done, shred the paper and throw it in the garbage, along with whatever food you were bingeing on.

Remember, this isn't about food. It's about control. It's about you losing control of yourself and doing something that feels safe—bingeing. Sure, you will pay for it later but right now you have to do it, don't you? You have to do something to show your anger and hurt feelings and frustration and bingeing is the only way you know how.

Food is the only thing you control: "I'll eat as much as I want and I'll show 'em!" You're not showing anybody anything. You are only hurting yourself. When you do this, you are not taking responsibility for yourself. You are letting others control you. You're saying to your body, "You're not good enough and I'm going to make you fat and unattractive."

Start today and take control of your food. Eat only what your body needs in order to fuel itself.

This holds try for *casual eaters* as well. These types of eaters will grab a bag of chips and, as they're reading or whatever, they will "casually" eat the entire bag before they know it. (Maybe just stop buying them altogether so they're not easily available.) My mom does this. She's a chip addict. She can't read a book or watch TV without a bag of chips at her side. Then she wonders why she can't lose weight.

If you do this, it's easier to break than bingeing. Just stop doing it. Whenever you find yourself reaching for your favorite casual food, stop mid-reach and close the cabinet door. Ask yourself, "Why am I doing this? I just ate a few hours ago. I need to stop casual eating." As with overeating, this is just a habit. You have to now teach yourself new, healthier habits.

And then there are the *Midnight Snackers*. These people actually get up in the middle of the night to eat! I have a close friend who does this. I asked her why and she said, "Because I'm hungry."

No, she isn't hungry. She's just gotten into the habit of doing it.

You shouldn't be doing anything at night but sleeping. (Unless you work third-shift.) If you find yourself wandering into the kitchen late at night, recognize that if you eat, you are going to gain weight and that's just that much more you have to lose. So, stop yourself, promise to have a good breakfast and go back to bed.

Or, when you wake up at night and start to get out of bed to do this: Just tell yourself no, roll back over and close your eyes. *Do not get out of that bed to eat!*

If you can break the habit just one time, you are going to be ahead of the game, folks. Just one time and the next time it will be easier not to give in. Soon, you'll have the habit broken all-together.

For some of you, you might have to do this on an hour by hour basis until you break your addiction and get over your feelings of boredom and frustration. Take as long as you need to take.

I don't think food addiction is much different than any other addiction. It's just legal. It makes you feel weak and sad and alone. You feel like you're the only person in the world who has ever been through this. You're not, I assure you. But you are fighting your own, unique struggle right now and it's a fight you have to fight on your own. And you will win. You will come out of the other side of it a better person. But you have to face up to it. You have to admit you have a problem.

If you struggle with this, go read a book or take a walk or a long, hot shower. Do anything to get your mind off food. Once you can conquer this, the rest is easy.

In review:

✓ If you are bingeing, why not sit down and write out your frustrations instead of eating?

✓ No one controls you but you. And only you can control your bingeing.

✓ If you are casual eating, catch yourself and put a stop to it. Casual eating is just a habit.

✓ Midnight snacking can be stopped. Just stop doing it!

✓ Form newer, healthier eating habits.

Weird places I lost weight.

As you lose weight, you will begin to notice that you are losing it in strange places. I did. And the strangest place of all was in my feet.

When I was gaining weight, I noticed that I was going up in shoe size. My feet just kept getting bigger and bigger and I went from a size seven and a half to a size nine and a half. In my feet! They didn't get longer, they got wider.

That was weird.

After I lost my weight, I noticed my shoes didn't fit like they used to. The good thing was that I got to buy new shoes! The bad thing was that I had just bought a pair of good sandals that set me back a few bucks. Because of the weight loss in my feet, I could no longer wear them.

Losing my chubby feet was more than worth a pair of sandals though. Unfortunately, along with my shoe size, my bra size went down, too. Sometimes, life just isn't fair.

Once you start to lose weight, you will notice that it comes off in weird places, like around your knees. Also, sounds strange, but your belly button will shrink in size. How weird is that? I know one person who told me that they had lost weight in their...shall we say, *nether regions*.

The best place it comes off is in your face. I look back at pictures of myself when I was overweight and think, "Good Lord, is that me?" My cheeks were so puffy, it looked like I had gauze stuck in them. And I had two chins. I was so happy when the second one disappeared.

So, look forward to all the good changes coming your way. Just know it's going to happen if you stop overeating. This should be more than enough incentive to get you on the right path.

And you might even get to purchase a few new pairs of shoes.

My current weight: 130 pounds.

That's what I now weigh. I am five-foot-three and weigh 130 pounds. I did have a goal to get down to 120 pounds, the weight I was at when I started college. I have done everything in the world to get down that low, but besides starving myself and not eating anything, there's nothing I can really do. Besides, when I weighed that much, I was only seventeen and wasn't fully developed.

Maybe the reason I "can't" get down to 120 is because I have a lot of muscle from working out. Even though my weight plateaued at 130, I continued to get thinner and thinner and my dress size got smaller and smaller. (Working out will do that because you reshape your entire body through exercise.)

Whatever the reason, I don't care. I'm happy here at 130. Sometimes the scale hits 128. That always makes me smile, but the next day, it might be at 131 or go up to 135. I once got down to 124, but I was sick during that time, so it came right back.

Eventually, I realized that our bodies are biologically programmed for a certain weight. Sure, I could do something drastic to lose those last ten pounds, but I don't want to. I feel fine like this and I can fit into a size six and, depending on the designer, sometimes a size four. One day I tried a pair of stretch pants on in a size two and they fit! They didn't look good, but they fit. Other times, I have had to wear a size nine and my favorite pair of shorts, though baggy, are a size ten.

You do understand that clothing size is arbitrary, don't you? One size *never* fits all.

So, the magical number of 120 just isn't coming around for me. If it did, I might look somewhat emaciated. I am happy with this weight. I do have to work at it in order to keep it and that's because I still continue to eat my favorite foods. Anyone can get skinny on lettuce sandwiches but, as I've said, I like food.

One thing you can do when you first start losing weight is to set yourself a weight goal. And, no, do not set yourself a weight goal of 120 pounds. Why? Because then you'd be setting yourself up for failure.

A suggestion: The first stage is around twenty pounds. Say you're a woman of average height and you weigh 200 pounds. (Obviously, the ratio will be different for men. Adjust accordingly.) You should set your goal at around 180 pounds. That's twenty pounds and a good amount of weight to lose. It may take a few months to do this, too. And, please note, if you don't lose it in a few months, you are not a loser. You just need to try a harder. *You will have to put some effort into this.* If you put no effort into it, nothing good will happen.

So, you get down to 180. Not too shabby. Now, how about going for 170? Take your time and enjoy the changes that are going on with your body. Enjoy life while it's going on, too. Don't stop everything just to lose weight. Continue to live and to work and to play.

Now that you've hit 170, how about going for 165? You might surprise yourself and go down to 160. Okay, and now you're 160, then how about 150? You can do it. You've come this far, haven't you? Now you're at 140, do you want to get down to 130? If so, keep it up. Eventually, your body will catch up to itself and it will get down to that weight it is supposed to be at. If you set too big a goal at once you are much more unlikely to achieve it.

That's what I did. I weighed 165. I said, "If I can get down to 150, I'll be fine." Once I got to 150, I thought, "Why not shoot for 140? I'll be *very* happy with that." Once I got to 140, I didn't even set a goal. But once I got to 130, I wanted to go for 120. Now I'm back to being happy at 130.

You will lose the most weight in the smallest amount of time. That means, you'll hit 165 sooner than you'll hit 130. And once you hit your "ideal" weight, the pounds will come off slower and slower. This is natural. Don't give up! You will plateau. And when you plateau, ask yourself what one food you can give up to get yourself over that hump. This doesn't mean you have to give it up indefinitely, it just means that you need to give it up until hit your weight goal. And the great thing is, once you give it up for that little amount of time, you probably won't want it anymore. And if you do want it, you will only want it sporadically.

Also, those last "ten" pounds are the hardest to lose. Most people I know are still trying to lose that last ten. If you "can't" lose them, do not beat yourself up. Just keep trying.

Again, your body is biologically programmed to be at a certain weight. It knows its ideal weight so if you get down to 130 or 135 or 140 or whatever pounds and the scale won't budge, then that's where you're supposed to be. When you find your ideal weight, just continue doing what you're doing. You don't have to change your eating patterns again.

So what if you do this and you don't lose any weight? This means you're not trying hard enough. You're not cutting back and more than likely, you're still snacking. Don't lie to yourself, either. If you do not expend any effort, you won't ever lose the weight. You have to make a concentrated effort to get the pounds off. If you "can't" do it, then try harder. Don't give up. If you relapse and go back to eating what you did before you began this weight loss plan, just start a new day today. Eventually, if you stick with it, you will lose the weight. But you have to make the effort. You have to apply yourself. You have to be willing to change your eating patterns. You can do it but you have to make a commitment to doing it.

Does this sound too simple to you? If it does, you need to have a little faith. All I know is that I am just a normal person and this is what worked for me. I hope it can work for you, too. Have faith in yourself that you can do it. I know how hard it is. I also knew that once I hit 165, it was only a matter of time before I tipped the scales at 200. It is so easy to gain weight and so hard to lose it. But if you change your eating patterns, you can do it. Nothing can stop you but yourself.

I am a work in progress and I will always look at myself as a work in progress. I don't limit myself at any certain point. I just know what I have to do to fuel my body and to make it look as good as it can be.

If you look at it like this and stop beating yourself up for not being "perfect", you will lose the weight. It's only a matter of time before you do.

In review:

- ✓ Set yourself a weight loss goal, beginning at around twenty pounds. Continue to do this until you have lost all the weight you want to lose.
- ✓ Know you will hit a weight-loss plateau. Do your best to get over that hump.

The scale is your buddy.

They say to throw away your scale. *They* say you shouldn't weigh but once or twice a week. *They* say the weight on the scale doesn't mean diddly-squat.

They are wrong.

How are you going to know if you're losing weight if you never weigh yourself? You're not. The scale is nothing but a tool for you to use while you are losing weight, and then to use to help you maintain it.

Go out and buy yourself a good scale. Now step on it. Don't cry and don't pout and certainly don't kick the dog. Face up to it. This is you and this is how much you weigh. Then check it just about everyday.

What I do is simple. I weigh everyday and try to keep my weight right around 130. If I see I'm gaining any weight, I cut back on my food intake. Obviously, I don't check it while I'm on vacation.

I weigh right when I get up in the morning. You can weigh at that time or at night, but I prefer the morning. I believe it to be the most accurate indicator of my real weight.

In review:

- ✓ Buy a good scale.
- ✓ Weigh yourself each day to check your progress.
- ✓ Don't freak out if you go up a little at first. Hold tight, it will go down soon enough—*if* you stop overeating, that is.

Warning! Don't double up!

If you heed my advice, you will lose weight. However, if you double up—eating more than a small plate of food—at supper time, you won't. Don't double up. Just think, "I know I'm a little hungry now and that's a good thing. That means this is working for me. Tomorrow, I promise, I will eat whatever I want for lunch. But right now, I have to be strong and have willpower. If I can get though this one night, I can make it the rest of the way."

Many nights, I go to bed a little hungry. When I wake up in the morning, I'm usually *never* hungry. I take this to mean that my body is fueling itself with the calories I stored yesterday. This is how I know it's working. Try it once and see. You'll be amazed at the results.

Eating at night will never help you to lose weight. That goes double for snacking. If you can cut these two things out, you're half-way there.

It's not going to happen overnight, but rest assured, it will happen. You just have to believe in yourself. Stop beating yourself up over the past. That's done and finished. Concentrate on today and what you can do to make the rest of your life better.

Remember, sometimes you are your own worst enemy. So start being your own best friend today.

In review:

- ✓ Do not double up at supper. By doubling up, I mean eating extra food that you know you don't need. You might feel hungry but that's because you're cutting back. "Hungry" doesn't mean you have to eat more than you should. Hungry means eat until you are satisfied.
- ✓ Do not eat at night.
- ✓ Do not snack.

The bread basket.
And other things to avoid in restaurants.

Have you been to a restaurant lately? They always bring you a basket of bread, don't they? And that bread usually has some kind of butter on it—honey butter usually—that melts along the top. The bread in those baskets is scrumptious. It's hard to resist. However, that little basket is causing a lot of people a lot of pain.

Bypass the bread basket. Go as far to tell your waitress you don't want it at your table. If it's not in front of you, you can't eat it. If she puts it down anyway, send it back with her.

There are other "little" things you can do that will save you plenty of calories. And it doesn't affect the taste of your food at all. Your belly just won't be as bloated.

With French fries, lay them on a napkin then put another napkin on top of them and squeeze out the oil. (Squeeze gently!) This saves bunches of calories and doesn't affect the taste at all.

In fact, you can do this with most greasy foods and, as I've said, it doesn't affect the taste one bit. Unless, of course, you like eating grease.

Most pizza has oil on the top, especially if it's a meat pizza. Take a napkin and dab the oil off. Don't squeeze, though, because you will squeeze the tomato sauce out.

You can also ask for extra ice in your sodas or tea and that saves calories. The ice melts and makes it yummier. Or you could take it a step farther and just drink water.

Never get a "to go" cup of soda or tea. This really adds up as well. Just toss it in the garbage after you're finished eating.

Potato chips are the worst things. They are empty calories. If you can avoid eating any chips, you are going to lose weight. I only eat chips a few times a month, if that much. I could never give up French fries but giving up chips was a lot easier for me.

When you get a cheeseburger, they usually put way too much mayo on it, don't they? Ask for mayo on the side and then put a little on yourself. You can even go as far to ask for all condiments on the side—mustard, ketchup, horseradish, etc. Also, always order salad dressing on the side. That way you can dip your veggies into it and get the most taste.

Croutons are a huge waste of calories. And they're also so hard they almost break your teeth off when you bite into them. What I do is take them off my salad and put them on a napkin. Why eat something that doesn't really have a taste and could send you to the dentist?

One more thing. Watch out for popcorn and all that other stuff at movies. I just bypass it on my way in. You should, too. You're treating yourself by seeing a movie and that's enough. However, if you can't resist the popcorn, get a small and don't get it drenched in butter.

In review:

- ✓ Decline the bread basket.
- ✓ When you eat fries, get a few extra napkins and slightly squeeze them so the grease will come off.
- ✓ Ask for extra ice for your drinks—or just drink water.
- ✓ Don't take your soft drink with you "to go".
- ✓ Try and delete chips from your meals.
- ✓ Ask for all condiments and salad dressings on the side.
- ✓ Don't buy movie popcorn. If you have to have popcorn, wait until you get home and pop some in the microwave that isn't loaded with all that heavy butter. (This will also save you tons of money.) Or, if you have to have one, get a small with no butter.

Another word on carbs.

I know most of us have tried this "miracle" diet where you eliminate all carbs from your diet. It has been my experience that this is just not a good idea.

The thing with carbs is that you *do* need them for your body. It's just that you don't need as much as you think you do. Carbs fill us up, but it's not a satisfying full. An hour or two later, you're hungry again—for more carbs. On that note, I do think we eat way too many carbs. But the carbs in veggies and fruits are good for you. Those things have minerals and vitamins that our bodies need and crave. All other carbs make us want more and more of them and they're not doing our bodies any good.

But we can't just give everything up, can we? I couldn't. I like eating cereal and popcorn. I also like my chips and salsa. Again, in moderation, carbs can be okay for your body. But only in moderation. If you eat a loaf of bread everyday, you are never going to lose weight.

Are you really hungry?

How to tell if you're hungry:
- ✓ Belly feels empty.
- ✓ You are lightheaded and bumping into stuff.
- ✓ You have no energy and can't concentrate.
- ✓ You have a headache.
- ✓ Belly hurts a little.
- ✓ Sounds of hunger erupting from belly.

Here's how to tell if you're not hungry:
- ✓ You just ate.
- ✓ You saw a cinnamon roll and your mouth watered.
- ✓ A sudden urge to chew. (Get some gum or a toothpick!)
- ✓ You want to eat because of lack of sleep. You could be tired. (Take a nap instead of eating.)
- ✓ You want to eat because you might be sad or angry.
- ✓ You want to eat because your taste buds are wreaking havoc inside mouth. Chew gum instead.
- ✓ You have any doubt that you're hungry. This means you're probably not hungry!

Home for the holidays.

During that time of the year, expect to gain a few pounds. I do. Everyone does. You can't help it. People are force-feeding you everywhere you go. You have parties at the office and at home. In the mall they're giving away free cookies and it's just hard not to indulge.

So, go ahead and eat an extra piece of pumpkin pie. Just know that you will have to lose it later on. If you're willing to make that commitment for eating that extra slice, go for it. But if you renege on your promise, you're only hurting yourself. (If a person wants to indulge with desserts, they should cut back on their meals during this time.)

People are so happy when they first lose weight, but then the holidays come up and they end up regaining. Not to worry! The trick is to go back to what you were doing *before* the holidays. The real challenge is making a commitment to keeping it off.

Remember the guidelines. They apply to holiday eating as well. And what are the guidelines?

Here you go:
- ✓ *Eat three meals a day.* A small breakfast, a moderate-sized lunch and small supper. You can do this during the holidays, too. Just don't overload your plate and don't ask for seconds.

✓ ***Don't snack.*** If you find yourself snacking on holiday foods, stop. If you want a holiday snack, then you might consider cutting back your meals to make up for it.

✓ ***Find your food triggers and learn to control them.*** During the holidays, your triggers will be going into overtime. Be aware of this.

✓ ***Stop obsessing about food.*** It's hard not to obsess when you're faced with turkey with all the trimmings. Be aware of what you're putting on your plate. Eat only about half of it and refuse seconds. Chances are, you have another dinner to go to and will have to eat there as well.

✓ ***Never overeat.*** Eat only to satisfaction. During the holidays, you will have to make a special effort to do this.

The next step: Working out.

Before you begin any exercise routine, you will need to consult your doctor. He/she will need to give you the go-ahead.

When you start losing weight, you will want to get your body into shape. This is just a natural progression. Not only will this help you burn more calories but it will shape your body and make you look fantastic.

Please stop crying. I know you hate exercising. If it makes you feel any better, I hate it, too. But I also know that if I *didn't* do it, I would feel worse than if I did. (It's called exercise guilt.)

Do you have to work out in order to lose pounds by not overeating? No, you don't. It just makes it easier. It also makes your body look great but if you hate exercising, that's your choice. But don't you want a better looking body? Don't you want to go to the beach without jiggling all over the place?

It really and truly doesn't take much effort to work out. You will need about thirty spare minutes a day and four days a week. That is only TWO HOURS a week. Sure it's much more fun to sit in front of the TV but the TV won't make you pretty now, will it? If you can't miss your favorite TV shows, exercise in front of the TV. It doesn't matter as long as you're exercising.

Depending on how out of shape and how overweight you are, you will have to tailor your workouts to suit your body type. You will probably have to start slow. I did. And do not beat yourself up if you can't do it all. Do as much as you can. Stop when you feel winded. This, like losing weight, will take time. The key is to find out what works best for you.

Basic types of workouts:
- *Strength training:* Using weights to build beautiful muscles.
- *Pilate's.* Uses core muscles. You will need another person or a video to do these moves. They are tough and I don't know if I would recommend them for beginners.
- *Yoga.* Surely you know what yoga is. Okay—it's an old form of exercise that concentrates on poses that stretch your muscles and makes you limber. It also entails deep breathing and meditation. A nice way to exercise as it does "center" and "relax" you.
- *Cardio.* Running, biking, doing anything to get that heart rate going. If you dislike any of these things, why not crank up the stereo and dance around like crazy?

I work out four times a week. Every other day, I do about twenty minutes of cardio—elliptical trainer, running in place, jogging, whatever as long as it keeps my heart rate up. The other two days, I strength train for thirty minutes.

There are a ton of other programs out there but I think most of them are a little hokey. The best ones are usually the simple ones. Anything fancy is not only going to tire your body but your mind as well. And some of them want you to work out for over an hour! I don't like working out for over an hour! I'm sure you don't either. I think that's one reason people don't work out because they think it takes too long.

And remember, start out slow. Even if it's just five minutes a day. Do something—anything—to start working out. Doesn't matter what—at first. But as you build your strength, do know that it will take more to keep you in shape. That's because your body gets used to what you're doing and once it stops being difficult, you're not burning as many calories or building as much muscle.

In review:
- ✓ It's always a good idea to exercise.
- ✓ Talk yourself into two hours a week.
- ✓ Pick your favorite routine and get to it.
- ✓ See your doctor before you start so he can give you the greenlight.

One of the best things about losing weight: New clothes!

One of the best parts of losing weight for me was getting to buy new clothes. I have always loved shopping and when I bought my first "skinny" outfit, I was ecstatic. But what tickled me even more was being able to throw all my old clothes out of my closet.

As I cleaned out my closet, I was amazed at all the things I'd once worn. My mouth dropped at how big some of the clothes were. I actually had a dress that resembled a tent! My old jeans were huge and shapeless. My t-shirts were mostly "one size fits all". It was a joy to clean all that out and put in new clothes that not only looked better, but made me feel better about myself.

Some people like to keep some of their old clothes around as a reminder of what they used to weigh. I have pictures and I don't want to be reminded, sorry. If it's there, in my opinion, you will find a reason to use it. My recommendation is to discard it all. Throw it out once you've *under*-grown it! Reward yourself by getting stylish clothes that make you look and feel good.

Another thing I was happy to buy was a bikini. I hadn't had a bikini since I was fourteen. I didn't get another one until I was in my thirties. I, simply, didn't have the confidence to wear one. But a few years ago, I went shopping and saw this fabulous bikini. I told myself I shouldn't even try it on, that it would look horrible on me. However, I couldn't resist. I forced myself to try it on and it looked great! I bought it *and* I wore it.

I not only lost weight, but through exercise, I reshaped my body. I look better now than I ever did when I was younger. No, I'm serious, I do. My body is in better shape and I feel better than I did when I was younger. And that's a good feeling.

In review:

✓ Once you lose weight, buy a few new outfits and throw all your old stuff out. That way you won't be tempted to "grow" back into it.

Growing older and getting better.

As I've said, I look better now than I did when I was in my twenties. I am healthier, happier and thinner. Who says being young makes a person happy? I don't think that's true. I think as we get older, we accept more about ourselves and we feel better, too. Little, stupid things don't bother us as much. We laugh more and we love more and we realize that being young, while it was fun, was just a stepping stone to the fabulous people we are now.

If I lack self-confidence in anything, it's not in my body. It's the best it can be and the best I can make it and it's only getting better. By adding body confidence, I have raised my opinion of myself. Not because I am focusing only on the visual, but because I am focusing on inner as well. Before, all I wanted to do was look good. Now I look good and I can turn my attention to other things. I can study new things or do whatever I want to do. I can do anything I want because this one thing—my weight—doesn't control my life anymore. It's done, it's over. I can move on to bigger and better things.

And all I have to do is maintain it is to not overeat.

I have been doing this for about nine years. It was nine years ago when I took that hard look in the mirror and really saw myself. It took me a good two years to get all my weight off. I kept getting thinner and thinner and I never gave up. After I started exercising, my body began to change and I liked that. I got even thinner. Once I saw results, I *wanted* to continue to get them. They happened because I *made* them happen. I knew transforming my body was going to take time, so I took that time to invest in it. I'm not getting a new one, so I didn't have much choice.

I'll be honest, while, sometimes it was very frustrating for me, it hasn't really been that much work. All I have to do is keep a check on my weight and give myself two hours a week to exercise. That's nothing!

But sometimes I do feel inadequate. In today's world, we are bombarded with pictures of super-skinny people in magazines that, quite truthfully, make us feel like we could do a little better to look more like that. I know sometimes I feel it, even after all my hard work. But I also know I am the best I can be. I've always hated the fact that I have very muscular legs. It wasn't until recently when I received a compliment on them that I realized they weren't as vile as I had originally thought.

Perception is everything.

The media really does a number on us, doesn't it? We don't really see ordinary, average everyday people on commercials or in the movies. And none of them look like they have an ounce of fat on them.

Wake up and stop feeling bad. These actors have probably had liposuction or they've got an eating disorder to be that thin. They are so thin they look emaciated. To me, they just don't look healthy. I don't care what any of them say, to get that thin you are doing *something*. There are very few people that are that naturally thin. And they are so thin, it's sad. There's a joke that the reason all models are bitchy is because they're all hungry. It's a sad joke, isn't it?

Don't aspire to look like him or her, whoever they might be. You shouldn't be jealous of another's body type because that's just unreasonable. And being jealous of some super-skinny person is like being jealous of their plastic surgeon or their eating disorder. You *do not* want an eating disorder.

We need to move away from the belief that there is an ideal body type. There's not. What appeals to one person, another one doesn't like.

And there is no fountain of youth.

All of us want to hold onto our youths so much that we fight wrinkles and saddlebags like they were an invading army. And they are, in a way. We want to look young, even when we are old.

But as I've said, there are perks to getting older. And one of them is growing wiser and knowing that while we can't stay young, we can stay active and we can look our best. Growing older is a better option than the other option we have. At least we're still alive! Growing older is much easier if you're in shape and not carrying around a lot of excess weight. Grow old well.

You have to make yourself the best that you can be. That doesn't mean you have to make yourself look like someone else. So the next time you find yourself comparing your legs or whatever to that of a model or actor, remember that they had different parents than you. It's genetics mostly and it's as simple as that.

Stop comparing and if find you can't, stop looking at magazines if all they do is make you feel bad about yourself. Magazines should make us feel better, shouldn't they? They shouldn't prompt us to become jealous and insecure but somehow, they do. And the reason is, before you even picked that magazine up, you were jealous and insecure.

That magazine did nothing but bring that out in you. Maybe there is something in your past that happened to you that made you insecure. Maybe your mom or whomever told you were overweight or ugly. No, they shouldn't have done that but you know what? *They were wrong.* They didn't know not to say these things; they didn't know that it would make you feel bad for the rest of your life.

Don't let them win. Stop today and face your insecurity issues. I did. I knew a lot of my insecurity came from my sisters and brothers taunting me. It hurt then but it doesn't hurt now. I'm over it because I don't believe them anymore.

Recognition of the problem is a big part of solving it.

It sounds too easy, but it's true. We've all been told we're ugly or stupid or that we "don't matter" at some point in our lives. How we let it affect us is the key to how we live our lives. Don't live your life for your mom or for your teacher or for the media. Live your life for *you.* Lose the weight for you because *you* want to look and feel better. Stop making it so hard. Stop fighting yourself right now, this day.

And because I have insecurity issues, too, I know one reason you're afraid to lose weight and look good is because you don't feel it's your right. Other people are overweight. They can't look good, so why should you?

Am I right? I know I am. It's like we have to punish ourselves because of our insecurity. You think, S*o what makes me that special person to do this? What makes me so special that I can look like a model? What makes me so special that I can persevere and be one of the beautiful, thin people?*

For starters, because you have a brain and you know how to use it. Just know that everyone suffers from low self-esteem from time to time.

I'll be honest and tell you that after about six months of trying to lose weight, I almost gave up. I had had it. I didn't want to suffer anymore. What kept me going? I didn't like the way I looked. I didn't like what I had become and I knew if I kept it up, it would spiral out of control and then I would really be in trouble. Not only would I have to deal with insecurity issues, I would have to deal with things like diabetes and heart disease. By staying overweight you are jeopardizing your health each and every day. Don't be stubborn and don't sabotage yourself any longer. Let me tell you something, once you get diabetes, you've got it for good.

I have a good friend who is diabetic, mainly because she's overweight and eats way too much sugar. She always cleans her plate and she always has a diet soda in her hand. She's in her sixties and we've worked together for a long time. I've seen her struggle for years with this disease. I've seen her gorge on sweets like she couldn't get enough. I've seen her in pain. I've seen her misery and if anything kept me from gaining the weight back, her experience did. She takes pills everyday because of her eating habits. Ask yourself this: *Do I want to have to take a pill everyday for the rest of my life?* I don't and I don't know anyone that does.

Health is paramount. As long as you have good health, you are as lucky as you can be. Riches and fame mean squat if you don't have good health. Do you know how many sick people would give anything to be healthy? I'll tell you. All of them.

In review:

✓ There is no fountain of youth.

✓ Everyone suffers from low self-esteem from time to time, even models and actors. They are people, too, after all.

✓ Face any insecurity issues that you have.

✓ Be the best you can be. Always. Starting right here, right now. Make a promise to yourself. Stick to your promise.

What's your good thing?

Look in the mirror and pick out one thing you like about yourself. Go on now, don't be shy. Do you have pretty eyes? Do you have thin ankles? It can be anything. For me, I have a good butt. I work it out enough, and it looks better now than it did when I was younger.

What is your good thing? Find it, concentrate on it and smile because you've got the best one out there.

Will losing weight make you happy? I don't know. It didn't make me any happier but it did make me more comfortable with my body. And that was good enough.

I think we're all about as confused about happiness as we are about dieting. Happiness is not a state of nirvana. To me, it's about being in a good mood, feeling good about my state of mind and my body. Happiness is just going with the flow and not letting every little single thing in the world upset me.

Losing weight did set me on a path not only for bodily health but for better mental health as well. And having peace of mind is better than having a million dollars in the bank. Not that I would know what having a million dollars in the bank is like, but…

You know.

We set our goals so high that once we reach them, we think everything will fall into place and we will suddenly and miraculously, be happier. Then, when it doesn't happen, we get sad and depressed.

The thing is to never give up. Just pledge to lose ten of those pounds, then ten more and then go from there. Don't worry if you're not doing it "fast" enough. You're doing it at your own pace. Calm down and relax a little, would you? You're losing more than you would have otherwise, right?

And be happy about what you're doing. Be happy that you're even trying. No one can ever take that away from you. *No one.*

In review:
- ✓ Pick your best feature and be proud of it.
- ✓ Set realistic goals.
- ✓ Never, ever give up.

A few more guidelines to Losing weight.

I would like to say I hope you are on your way to a healthier, better life and I wish you the best of luck. I know how hard it is to lose weight. I know because I was there. I know sometimes I just wanted to give up and forget about it. But something spurred me on. The key is to find your something, whether it's wanting to be around for your kids or grandkids or taking that trip to Europe or just working in the garden. Whatever it is you want in your life, work towards that goal and the rest should fall into place.

Once you change your habits, you will change your life. I know everyone says this but it's true. You can do it and you can do it by just making the decision to do it. It is really all up to you. No one can do this for you; it's something you have to do for yourself.

One of the most important things I can say to you is this: Whatever your weight is right now, don't gain any more than that. If you never lose one more pound, just don't gain any more. That extra ten or twenty or one-hundred can easily turn into twenty or thirty or two-hundred. And that's because most of the foods in our lives are addicting.

However, food is only addicting if you let it be. It is not a drug and it does not have control over you. Recognizing this is paramount. It's one of the most important things you can do. Take control now and stop worrying about losing weight. Now I don't worry about it. I do keep it in check and I do watch what I put into my mouth, but if I gain a few pounds here or there, I know just to cut back for a few days and it usually comes right back off.

I just want to give you a few, simple guidelines to losing weight. You don't have to use all of them nor do you even have to use any of them. But if you keep this stuff in mind, it will make your weight loss experience all the easier.

Guidelines to losing weight:

- ✓ You have to want to lose weight and keep it off.
- ✓ You have to admit you're overweight.
- ✓ Pen the problems in your life, have a good cry, cleanse yourself.
- ✓ Write down what you eat, when you ate it and why. "Being hungry" is rarely the reason. "Boss upset me" is more likely.
- ✓ Keep a check on your eating habits. Are you eating at night? Are you snacking out of boredom? If so, find a new hobby, read a book or go for a walk.
- ✓ Donuts are evil! Just kidding. If you want a donut, have one donut and save the others for another time.
- ✓ Don't overeat at breakfast unless you plan on cutting back for the rest of the day. Breakfast should just be a little something to get you going.
- ✓ "Save" your calories for your one main meal during the day. I find it's best to eat this meal at lunch. During that meal, eat whatever you want. During dinner, have a bit less. Gradually you will want less and less food as your body grows tighter and your appetite diminishes in size.
- ✓ Don't skip meals.

✓ Never snack! If you do snack, only have a handful of raisins or a piece of fruit. Don't look at snacks as a reward. They aren't! They are only a way to keep you from losing weight.

✓ Drink eight glasses of water per day.

✓ If you're hungry mid-afternoon, take one bite of something and throw the rest away. Remember that dinner will here before two shakes of a lamb's tail!

✓ Ignore hunger if you have had your meals. It is all in your mind!

✓ Stop judging yourself. Don't say, "I'll never do it! Wah!" No, not with that attitude you won't.

✓ Commit! It took me two years to get the weight off. It may take you more or less. COMMIT to doing it and do it right this time!

✓ Have a goal of losing ten or twenty pounds. Set several small, attainable goals, rather than one large, intimidating one. After you lose it, set another goal and then keeping going until you are where you want to be, weight-wise.

✓ Don't starve yourself. You will only overeat later.

✓ Wait until you're hungry to eat and food will taste divine.

✓ Some days you will be hungrier than others.

✓ Keep a check on PMS. It makes you want salt and sugar like nobody's business.

✓ Don't eat because you think you'll be hungry later. Eat only when you *are* hungry.

✓ Don't eat because you feel "weak". Know this is probably all in your mind. See if it goes away and if not, you might want to see your doctor.

- ✓ Share a meal at a restaurant. We all know they want us to get our money's worth, so they overfeed us. Sharing a meal saves money, calories and bloat.
- ✓ Never eat in front of the TV, while reading or anything else. Enjoy your food. Eat at a table even if you're by yourself.
- ✓ Eat what you want. This includes all that terrible junk food. BUT only eat part of it. Never all of it.
- ✓ Keep in mind that the healthier you eat, the healthier you will be. So mix it up some and eat fresh vegetables and fruits and lean meats as well as the foods you like.
- ✓ Any food that goes in and isn't needed will end up on your body somewhere. Extra food is nothing more than storage.
- ✓ Never fool yourself into thinking that overeating/snacking when you're not hungry is excusable. It isn't. It will make you gain weight.
- ✓ Never clean your plate. No matter how good it is.
- ✓ Love yourself and your body. Know that you can change the shape of your thighs but you can't change your genetics. Learn to pick out your best attributes and focus on what is good about yourself, not what is "bad". "Bad" is all in your mind.
- ✓ *See a doctor before beginning this or any other program. I am not an expert. I'm just someone like you who got fed up with dieting.*

Congratulations! You've succeeded. Now what?

It was a lot of work, but it paid off, didn't it? You've lost the weight! Now the tough part. How do you keep it off? Is it going to be hard? Is it going to drive you crazy? No, not if you do what I do in order to maintain my weight.

The thing with my weight loss method is that you have changed your eating patterns. Once you do that and stop overeating and snacking, all you have to do is continue that. You can never go back to eating the way you did before, but that way got you into a lot of trouble, didn't it?

All you have to do now is have your three meals a day: One small breakfast, one moderate lunch and one small supper. That's it. If you continue this, you really shouldn't have to even worry about weight gain. Keep an eye on the scale, too. It's what's going to help you know when you gain a few pounds and when you do, all you have to do is cut back on your food intake.

Know that if you begin and stick to an exercise program, it's going to make all this much, much easier. You don't have to exercise, but it will make you feel better. And it will help you to maintain your weight.

Ladies and gentlemen, that's it. I'll shut up now.

In review:

- ✓ Once you've lost the weight, simply continue doing what you're doing.
- ✓ If you go up a few pounds, just cut back for the next few days and they should come right back off.
- ✓ Don't ever go back to eating the amount of food that you did when you were overweight.

Printed in the United States
127938LV00001B/18/A